T0194168

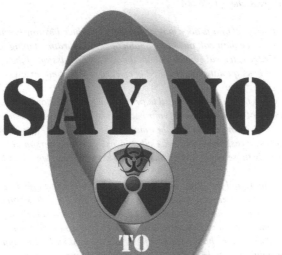

SAY NO

TO

Radiation and Conventional Chemo

Winning My Battle Against Stage 2 Breast Cancer

By

Diana Warren and Jamie Beardsley

Foreword By James W. Forsythe, MD, HMD

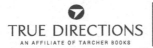 TRUE DIRECTIONS
AN AFFILIATE OF TARCHER BOOKS

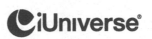 iUniverse®

SAY NO TO RADIATION AND CONVENTIONAL CHEMO
WINNING MY BATTLE AGAINST STAGE 2 BREAST CANCER

Copyright © 2014 Diana Warren.
Book Design by Patty Atcheson Melton.

All rights reserved. No part of this book may be used or reproduced by any means,
graphic, electronic, or mechanical, including photocopying, recording, taping or by
any information storage retrieval system without the written permission of the publisher
except in the case of brief quotations embodied in critical articles and reviews.

The information within this book is intended to provide helpful points of information should you
seek to become aware of more options for your health. The supplements, treatments, and nutrition
herein were successful for the author, but they may not be suitable for everybody. Everyone's
health requirements and response to various substances differ from person to person. The views
in this book are merely those of the author based upon her own experiences and research.

The researchers, author, and publisher are not responsible for the side effects, consequences,
or actions resulting from the treatments and supplements in this book. It is still advised
that you visit your own physician. The contents of this book are not a substitute for the
advice of a professional. If you think you have a health issue or emergency, please seek
medical help immediately. This book contains material protected under International
and Federal Copyright Laws and Treaties. Any unauthorized reprint or use of this
material is prohibited, under civil and federal and governmental penalties.

iUniverse books may be ordered through booksellers or by contacting:

iUniverse
1663 Liberty Drive
Bloomington, IN 47403
www.iuniverse.com
1-800-Authors (1-800-288-4677)

Because of the dynamic nature of the Internet, any web addresses or links contained in
this book may have changed since publication and may no longer be valid. The views
expressed in this work are solely those of the author and do not necessarily reflect the
views of the publisher, and the publisher hereby disclaims any responsibility for them.

ISBN: 978-1-4917-4426-0 (sc)
ISBN: 978-1-4917-4428-4 (hc)
ISBN: 978-1-4917-4427-7 (e)

Library of Congress Control Number: 2014914248

Printed in the United States of America.

iUniverse rev. date: 8/14/2014

DEDICATION

To Jamie Beardsley, my devoted, loving daughter and personal
angel; to Dr. Edward O. Terino, my longtime friend, Dr. John
Matrisciano, and Dr. James Forsythe. There are no words to thank
you all for what you've done for Jamie and I over the past years.
Your actions were valiant.

Contents

Forword
JAMES W. FORSYTHE, M.D., H.M.D.

Diana Warren's breakthrough book, *"Say No to Radiation and Conventional Chemo: Winning my Battle Against Stage 2 Breast Cancer"* delivers to breast cancer patients throughout the United States, as well as other cancer patients who are facing the ordeals of being diagnosed with this often deadly disease, from the perspective of a wise and proactive patient herself, with emphasis on taking control and being skeptical about conventional medicine. She steps out of the box to find the best "tailor-made" treatments available without falling into the complacency of treatment protocols offered by conventional medicine.

Breast cancer in the United States occurs in one out of eight women and is the second leading cause of death after lung cancer in the year 2013, surpassing 50,000 deaths per year. Diana's journey through conventional breast cancer "cookbook" programs is well chronicled, and the underlying angst that she relates is vividly portrayed in her account.

My input comes from being an integrative oncologist who has practiced conventional oncology alone for twenty of my forty years in medical practice. After graduating in the top twenty percent of my class at the University of California at San Francisco (at the time, one of the top five medical schools in the country), I have had experience as an army pathologist, as an emergency room physician, Internal Medicine-certified specialist, a geriatric physician with certification as director of more than six extended care facilities in Northern Nevada, a hospice director, an instructor an instructor of medicine at the University of California at San Francisco, and an associate professor of medicine at the University of Nevada at Reno Medical School. In addition, I am a Board-Certified Homeopathic physician, an author of more than twelve books and numerous chapters relating to various aspects of medicine, cancer care, and cancer politics.

Here are some examples of the many reactions I personally have witnessed directly from my patients in circumstances akin to what Diana describes in her tell-all ordeal with breast cancer. Once the word "cancer" is mentioned, patients often feel "blinded and deafened" by the word itself, and after anything is discussed beyond that point, it simply becomes a blur and is not absorbed. The cliché "I was a deer in the headlights" is commonly stated by patients and refers to the fact that they feel immobilized and can barely walk, think, or talk. They often describe being "numb and immobile". Multiple emotions come rushing forward. These emotions may be anger, confusion, fear, self-pity, feeling cheated, denial, overwhelming worry about other family members and their reactions, and the need to confide in close friends, as well as struggle to soak in the stigma of having a potentially fatal disease and what it all means. In regards to their professions, their retirement plans, their monetary resources and their general lifestyle, everything is on the table in terms of uncertainty. The feeling of hopelessness soon enters the emotional drama in regards to their marriage; being unable to see their children grow up, graduate, and achieve their professional goals; to see their grandchildren; and to contribute to their family's well being.

In those few minutes, hours, days, and weeks following their diagnosis, patients will experience physical symptoms such as dry mouth, rapid heartbeat, overwhelming fatigue, and decreased energy. In searching for educational resources, there is a feeling of mental gridlock with too much information available in magazines, medical books, and on the Internet. Support groups and other victims' personal accounts and recommendations are also sought after but seldom satisfy all of their needs.

Sometimes overwhelming panic and anxiety occur, causing insomnia, tremors, and an inability to organize thoughts.

Often times the attending oncologist or radiation therapist will amplify these conditions by telling the patient to get ready for becoming weak for further surgery, the beginning of radiation therapy and chemotherapy – either given concomitantly with the radiation therapy or to follow with radiation therapy. Then on top of all this, the patient has to hear of all the adverse reactions to the three major treatments. With surgery, it is the possibility of anesthetic complications and hospital-borne infections. With radiation therapy, it is the collateral damage to nearby organs such as the heart, lungs or skin. With chemotherapy, it runs the gambit from chemo brain to hair loss, nausea, vomiting, skin rashes, anorexia, cytopenias, infections, extreme organ damage, and even death.

Diana outlines all of these decisions in a very personal and poignant manner in order to help others undergoing the same trauma, and she brings it home in a very personal way. The major goal of this book is her skepticism with conventional medicine and distrust of the system, which, after one-hundred-billion dollars in taxpayer monies over a forty-year period, has given us essentially a defeat on the "war on cancer", as declared by the Nixon Administration in the early 1970s. By their own literature alone, Stage IV cancers after a five-year period of chemotherapy, both in this country and in Australia, can only achieve a 2.1 to 2.3 percent survival rate.

Diana was able to sift through the conventional dogma and decided to look for cutting-edge answers. To do this, she sought out second opinions from Integrative Oncology, a new and recognized field and subspecialty of standard Oncology. She was able to provide a positive opinion after studying genetic chemo-sensitivity testing and its value, which is often followed by insulin-potentiated therapy, which is low-dose and nontoxic. These modalities for the first time in a cancer patient's treatment protocol provide a blueprint to ensure a predictable high remission rate and takes the guess work and unpredictability out of the decision making. The follow-up treatment with insulin-potentiated therapy markedly reduces the high averse toxicity rate and sequelae that occur ever too frequently. Even death, if it occurs after the first course of full-dose chemotherapy, presents no liability for the oncologist or radiologist or surgeon as they are simply doing cookbook protocol treatments authorized by the National Cancer Institute.

Instead of buying into the recommendations given by her conventional oncologist, which would at best be a guessing game as to which toxic drugs to take and for how long, without truly knowing if any of the two or three drugs given to her would actually work to kill her cancer cells and stem cells, Diana instead chose genetic testing, which gives certainty to the decisions made in regard to the drugs used. Also, conventional medicine would more than likely want her to have radiation therapy after completing a four to six month course of chemotherapy. At that point, what are they treating? Are they treating normal breast tissue because tumor markers are normal? MRI scans, ultrasounds, and mammography studies are normal. So, in most cases they are treating normal breast tissue, but they are covering themselves with a large dose of radiation therapy, which only is going to impact their immune system in a negative way.

Therefore, in all of these decisions, Diana has made the right choice, and kudos to her for her courage in doing so.

This book is a "must read" for all newly diagnosed cancer patients and their families, and it is a courageous attempt by a single individual to record her trials and tribulations in making the decision she has made.

Get a Second Opinion

Jamie Beardsley

This is the story of my mother and her journey to healing. A prescription of conjugated estrogen tablets was given to her years ago and now the medication derived from the urine of pregnant mares had caught up with her. The label should have read, "Helps now, but may cause something bad later!" I know in my heart that those pills caused this cancer. She has always been into health and read everything there was on the subject. Smart, wise and knowledgeable are just some of her wonderful traits. This story begins when some discomfort came off and on in one side of her breast. Also really strange, every day and night my mom's cat curled up right next to her feet, almost as if the pet were trying to heal its owner. To say the least, I thought that was interesting.

Mother decided to see a doctor in Las Vegas. But he just said, "We'll keep an eye on it." Guided by her feelings, she questioned him and then decided to call another physician in California, Edward Terino, whom I consider one of the world's best doctors. She trusted him following a friendship of many years. He recommended that she visit Doctor John Matrciano. So it begins.

When my mother makes up her mind about something she becomes like an unstoppable freight train. Thank God, because of this characteristic mom played a pivotal role in eventually saving herself, determined from the start to "get this horrible thing"—the tumor—out of her as soon as possible. So, the day after speaking with Dr. John Matriciano, she drove to Thousand Oaks, California, to Doctor Matrciano's clinic for an examination. She felt happy after initially visiting Doctor Matrciano; that's when he removed the tumor. Other clinics or doctors' offices that my mother had previously visited had refused to remove the disease despite her assertions that the tumor should be removed as soon as possible.

Now, the hard part—waiting. Nothing is worse than sitting in a hotel room in steadily growing anticipation that someone soon would call with life-or-death news about your fate. Near mother in the hotel room, I watched mother as she spoke on the phone to her doctor. Her head drooped, a definitive signal to my heart that this was indeed bad news. When you're an only child, your mother your only living close relative, your world stops. My father was alive but had not been part of my life. By contrast, my mom had always been there for me, and she would do anything for me. The relationship I have with her is not like anything I can describe. When she hurts, I hurt. Words cannot describe my love for her.

After the shocking news, which took a full week to sink in, we both knew that we had to do something fast to heal her. As described by Doctor Matrciano, mother's cancer at the time was a at an aggressive Stage 2 level. He told her to get chemotherapy and gave her a plan. Well, my mother isn't one to follow the crowd. She always thought differently than everyone else. I'm like that, too.

She suffered horrible pain following the surgery. My heart broke when watching someone that I love so dearly suffer intense physical pain. I ran out for whatever she needed during our stay in the hotel room, determined to do everything I could to help alleviate her suffering. We wanted mother to return home, but for several weeks she needed to say in the hotel to remain close to the doctor. Helping my mother became all that mattered to me. I did everything possible to ensure that she was all right, striving my utmost to get everything that she needed.

Well, after we had spent nearly one month in the hotel mother proclaimed that she felt ready to return to Las Vegas. If mom had proceeded to follow Doctor Matrciano's recommendation, she would start chemotherapy treatments near her Southern Nevada home.

Mother's situation got interesting again; her physical condition remained fragile, making her sore and not feeling healthy enough to drive herself. From mom's house, I gave her a ride to a medical facility that she had found. A wave of strange vibes engulfed me as I sat in the complex's parking lot, waiting for mom to return to my vehicle from her first chemotherapy treatment. While still alone in my car and waiting, intuition told me that mother did not want to be there, that something "was going wrong." Indeed, momentarily she returned to our vehicle. Initially she refrained from saying anything.

"I never, ever want to go back there," mother eventually said as I drove her home, a stunned expression that I had never before seen embossed on her face. "Everything in there looks gray, so bad that it scares me."

Invariably, I eventually learned that mother returned to the same clinic three additional times. But in every instance she refrained from undergoing chemo.

To her great credit and once again showing her strong will and tremendous determination, mother declared to me that she would never subject her body to such poisons—declaring that "there has to be something better."

From that point forward, mother dove into a full-scale investigation, more determined than ever to discover a healthy, effective, non-toxic treatment.

Increasingly determined to save her own life, she scoured the Internet while reading everything possible to find a reliable, non-poisonous cure. My respect and admiration for her multiplied as she refused to accept the universal declaration by standard-medicine doctors that enduring chemo is the accepted protocol, the universal "standard of care."

Perhaps predictably, at least when accounting for her superior intellect and take-charge attitude, mother was not going to accept a potentially fatal treatment just because some medical professional told her to do so.

Mother allowed her instincts to serve as her guide, launching a quest for a second opinion. For my part, I remained determined to do whatever I could to help, willingly putting my life "on hold" thanks to my unbending love for her.

In a sense some observers might say that I became her mother, wanting to always be there to help, to relieve her of all pain and to make her feel better in any way possible.

A realization emerged. I had become the only person that my mother felt she could depend on besides herself. More than ever as the weeks and months steadily passed I became increasingly determined to prevent anything from stopping me from helping her get well. Essentially I evolved into mother's full-time nurse, a task that I loved.

She made the best of her rest time, seizing that as an opportunity to continue her relentless, non-stop Internet-based quest to pinpoint an ideal natural, non-poisonous treatment option. On days when she felt strong and good enough, she seized those moments to resume her vital quest to find the best information. Certainly by this point in life I had already become fully cognizant of mother's unstoppable fortitude. Nevertheless, I began feeling truly amazed upon witnessing an ill person of her small physical stature using mostly her will and determination to locate vital healing alternatives. Mom's doctors eventually admitted their amazement, impressed at the amount of critical information that she had discovered.

Eventually she began to identify non-toxic herbs that some practitioners of homeopathic or natural medicines deemed helpful for her type of breast cancer. At this juncture although unsure of how such substances might taste or how she might get them, in her mind anything was better than the horrors she had witnessed at the chemo treatment centers.

Thanks to her research, mom learned why homeopaths insist that sugar serves a perhaps one of the worst and most deadly triggers in causing or igniting cancer. Determined to help her find viable foods, I decided to visit a health food store in hopes of locating a viable, non-cancerous sugar-free alternative. Mother had determined that many sugar substitutes including saccharine are suspected carcinogens.

Thanks to my own tenacity, similar to mother's in many ways, at a Whole Foods store I found amazing drops comprised of stevia, a healthy, non-toxic plant substance that many people consider just as sweet as sugar. I bought samples from a wide variety of stevia-droplet flavors, before soon encouraging mother to taste them to determine which she liked most.

Just as impressive, I also discovered that stevia can help mask the bland tastes of certain herbs or plants deemed effective by homeopaths in the treatment of and the prevention of certain cancers. Meantime, via mail-order, mom had purchased numerous herbs and foods that she deemed as potentially helpful in her overall treatment regimen. Increasingly eager to help make life easier and better for her, I went on many adventures to retrieve her orders from the mailbox.

Although her body rejected or disagreed with some of these substances, other foods seemed to work wonders in advancing her overall recovery. An added responsibility emerged for me, a critical need to regularly ensure that she took the right substances in proper amounts at specific, pre-set times. Sensing the importance of these essential tasks, I made sure to tell her every day not to forget anything.

Her healing continues.

Needless to say, mother's journey back toward optimal health has taken a very long road and today she is doing great, increasingly determined to tell the whole world of the vital importance of getting a second opinion.

To me this proverbial beacon of light, this proverbial torch that my mother carries in striving to bring this message to the entire world, also illuminates the fact that she shall eternally hail as my favorite person in the whole world—as I continue loving her with all my heart.

Part I
My Own Path

Chapter 1
A Long-Standing Mistrust

My mistrust of medical facilities, doctors and treatments began at a very early age. Most of my relatives understood healthcare. My mother and grandmother were nurses, and my grandfather a doctor.

I was born Diana Rosslyn shortly before World War II in Santa Monica, California, to a mother and father who had just said their marital vows a few days earlier. I'm unsure how or when they met, but their romance carried them all across the U.S., and all throughout their lives. My mother was carefree and adventurous, taking social drinking to a higher level.

She was born Walta Irene Anderson in Dalhart, Texas. She had one older sister, a younger brother, and a busy life with hard-working and nurturing parents. Mother loved animals, music, art, traveling, adventures and men. Her father, George M. Anderson, was a violin maker with clients from many countries. I know this because my mother saved a small album with his pictures and letters. My favorites include a tiny postage stamp-sized card where George wrote the Ten Commandments on that small space.

My maternal grandmother, Allie Taylor Anderson, always believed that everyone in the family needed to work. Allie and George lived in Dalhart, rearing their three children until George became ill following a trip to Europe delivering a couple of custom violins. He died within a few months and Allie packed up her three young children with what belongings fit into her old car and drove to Glendale, California.

Grandma Allie rented a home located at 1125 East California Street. Her business card read: "Mrs. Allie Anderson's Private Hospital."

I don't know the year of their move, but my mother must have been about 10 years old. By keeping all three youngsters—one of whom was my mother—in one bedroom, Grandmother Allie was able to rent out the other rooms for "rest home care."

Determined to find a better place to live and work, my grandma decided to leave Glendale. She immediately leased the former Hollywood home of old stage and film character actor Taylor Holmes, perhaps most famous for his portrayal of Marilyn Monroe's father-in-law in the 1953 film "Gentlemen Prefer Blondes."

Allie became determined to increase her income, convinced that Hollywood was full of people that wanted her services. Correct in this regard, she amassed a waiting list for "residents." Some were writers, others artists of paint and music. Grandma served the colorful residents breakfasts and dinners in a large oval dining room that opened to gardens, winding walkways and a fish pond. The home featured many patios and private nooks to rest, everything located in the shadow of the famed Yamashiro Building at 1999 N. Sycamore Avenue in Hollywood.

During its 99 years since being build in 1914, the Yamashiro has emerged as a historical landmark. The building has witnessed the birth of the film industry, the glamour of Hollywood's "Golden Age," the difficult times of war with Japan and Germany, and the current period of intense interest in Eastern cultures. Yamashiro started as a fabulous private estate and is now open to the public, widely acclaimed for its unique restaurant and lavish public gardens.

Yamashiro means "Mountain Place" in Japanese. It was the dream of the Bernheimer brothers in 1911 to build a hilltop mansion 250 feet above Hollywood Boulevard, an ideal structure to house their priceless collection of Asian treasures. The brothers brought hundreds of skilled craftsmen from the Orient to recreate the exact replica of a palace located in the "Yamashiro" mountains near Kyoto, Japan. The siblings made their dream a reality.

I must confess that as children my friends and I went to Yamashiro and played on the black shiny floors, all of us fascinated by the furnishings. We were usually chased out by a few claps and laughter.

My well-meaning Grandmother Allie enrolled me in dance school. I took a few dancing lessons from movie star legend Rita Hayworth's uncle, Jose Cansino. His school was on La Brea near Hollywood Boulevard, a few steps from the famous old Sartu Theater. Later while in high school I briefly worked at the theater and enjoyed many exciting nights seeing various movie stars as they watched the plays.

My dance lessons were few since I never remained in one place for very long. For the same reason I also missed out on my piano lessons.

As many people today can very well imagine, Hollywood was indeed a very exciting place during the 1940s.

People would talk about the Macambo Nightclub, Ciero's, and the Garden of Allah on Sunset Boulevard, a hangout of the stars. Down the street was Schwab's drug store where Lana Turner had been "discovered." So many others flocked there to sit at the same famous soda fountain. My grandmother and I often would walk up and down Hollywood Boulevard for an exciting afternoon or evening.

There would be all kinds of goings on. Among just a handful of examples: a man sold gardenias from a tray trapped around his neck; and a dwarf with no legs on a square skateboard sold newspapers. It was always different, and at that time very safe. The small shops kept busy with pedestrian traffic, and there were no parking meters anywhere.

Grandmother Allie continued to serve as my strength, always there through the chaos for me with unquestioning love.

My mother had left home to be on her own about the age of 16 to work in the nursing field and to seek excitement. Mom had a brief marriage that resulted in a stillborn boy, promptly told by physicians after this personal tragedy that she could have no other children.

I don't know where or how my parents met, but when they did, it was passionate and exciting.

My father, Edward Rosslyn, was the only son of native Romanians, Doctor Isadore Marcu and Sophie Rosslyn. Grandfather Isadore's school papers are dated 7th of July (Julie) 1903 from a medical facility in Romania. I don't know anything about grandfather's life until he immigrated to the United States. I was told that when unrest began across Europe before the outset of World War I, this grandfather—often affectionately called "Doc"— took Sophie and made the trip to Chicago. En route they went through the famed Ellis Island with so many others.

Their Certificate of Naturalization is dated 10 of December, 1914. Isadore was 27 years old and Sophie 27. The certificate also indicated that the couple "resides with one minor child of five years of age, Edward. Address is 3515 W. 12th, Chicago, Illinois."

The couple eventually became U.S. citizens following several years of study.

Grandfather Isadore's Romanian medical documents were translated and certified in Chicago, which allowed him to practice medicine. He continued schooling in order to fulfill the needs of patients who required dental and prosthetic care. To his credit, while living in a railroad car that he had "fixed up" for his family, grandfather completed courses at the Chicago College of Dental Surgery in May 1907. They were later able to afford a tiny apartment and Sophie gave birth to a daughter, June Rosslyn. Sadly, she died of breast cancer at age 43 in about 1956.

At some point in time Doc and Sophie moved to Los Angeles, where he continued to treat patients in hospitals and from home. He never felt the need for an office.

Wise and money conscious, Grandfather Isadore invested his earnings in mid-size apartment houses in the Silver Lake neighborhood near downtown Los Angeles, and in other mid-LA neighborhoods.

A frugal and crafty spendthrift, Doc never purchased a traditional home. He felt that an apartment was just fine, especially if you owned it along with the building's 30 other units. I often stayed with my Grandma and Grandpa Rosslyn at their various properties, discovering that you can quickly skate in and out of older elevators. Funny, I still have one of my skate keys; no one I know has any idea what this is.

All of Doc's life he practiced mixing medicine with common-sense cures. He continued to make house calls in Los Angeles to the day that he died in the late 1950s.

Needless to say, Grandfather Isadore was a great contributor to my passion for investigating and questioning generally accepted methods and what was being taught. He had a delicious sense of humor and often played jokes on his family members. I remember saying goodbye to him at Los Angeles International Airport in the early '50s, as he departed for France on a TWA plane that had three tails. Everyone in my family became worried whenever he made a long trip, all of them terrified of flying. Doc made several trips to Europe and always returned safe. Yet my father never flew on a plane.

Grandfather Isadore's loving wife, my Grandmother Sophie, outlived him by 10 years and remained a kind, silent woman until her death. She never drove a car, flew in an airplane or wore pants, always dresses.

My father Edward Rosslyn studied in Chicago at Northwestern and that's all I know about him until he married my mother a few days before I was born. Trouble erupted and continued from the start of their young marriage. Mother was reared an Irish Catholic, a sharp contrast to father's lifestyle from a Romanian Jewish family. Neither parent followed or practiced either of their religions as adults. The in-laws remained in a constant uproar most of the time.

My parents decided that they could work together owning and running a sanitarium, boosted by experience and knowledge honed from their separate but fairly similar backgrounds. Doc loaned them funds to purchase Mount Gleason Sanitarium in Sunland, California. My folks brought me there to live as a baby.

Looking back today, odd memories float to the surface of my mind. The most memorable characters included Barbara, a bizarre old patient who tiptoed around the patio area. (She is featured in the photo section of this book; she's the tall person wearing a robe in a photograph of nurses and patients.) The woman would grunt sometimes carrying a trashcan while looking for something.

One day while shaded by overhead grapevines hanging from a trellis, Barbara looked in her trashcan and grunted. Curious, I went over and peaked inside. I saw a long speckled length of scales, a large rattlesnake that Barbara had captured.

The hospital staff quickly killed and buried the snake. They were always warning us to remain on the lookout for such creatures. The sanitarium's personnel and residents often encountered rattlers, coyotes and deer that had ventured from the surrounding hillsides.

Another of my disturbing memories involved a patient whose agonizing howls and screams erupted early one morning. Her gown had somehow caught fire, ignited by a floor heater—before the woman ran down a hallway while engulfed in flames.

The nurses and my mother caught the woman, wrapped her in blankets and rolled her on the floor.

Ghost hunters today still say that some of the deceased patients continue haunting Mount Gleason Sanitarium.

When World War II erupted I remember hearing the initial details with family and friends while sitting around a radio. I failed to understand what was happening but everyone became upset while some cried.

Now all of our lives were going to change and disruptions would be the norm.

Drafted right away, my father became convinced that my mother could manage Mount Gleason during his absence while serving as a soldier. Our family realized that my young mother faced a formidable challenge in managing a full sanitarium without father's support. I doubt they could foresee the strain that this decision would put on all of us.

Mother spent long hours working valiantly pushing herself to the limits. I was told later that she had curbed her drinking while really doing a stupendous job. Determined to earn as much as possible, she took extra shifts at local hospitals whenever such opportunities emerged. Many hospitals during that period were short-handed, while lacking the type of stringent government-imposed restrictions enforced today.

"What a shift! I'll be darned if the doctor wasn't near drunk and two of his nurses smelled like they joined in, too. I was the only one who had any sense today."

She witnessed many errors at the hospital, and as a result became increasingly jaded. Aware of how such negligence and malpractice could impact her loved ones, mother imparted a lesson to me that I never forgot.

"Diana," she said, stooping down and placing her hands on my little shoulders, her impassioned dark eyes staring at me. "I want to tell you something. If you are having an operation, mark that area yourself with a pen. Understand all the meds you are given before you take them. People die in hospitals due to careless mistakes."

The terror of that possibility stuck with me at the impressionable age of four.

My young mother found herself wanting more pleasures in life. She began working too hard at nursing while also managing Mount Gleason.

Apparently mother had grown weary of my father's absence and his letters from different locations in the U.S. She became interested in our new produce delivery man, Sol, a strong, blond, blue-eyed polish gent who delivered our orders twice weekly.

Sol had two brothers. The youngest, Bennie, collected bugs, beetles and butterflies from around the world. Somewhat gross-looking due primarily to his bad teeth, Bennie often scared me with his giant beetles. I sometimes watched him stick pins in the butterflies before placing them in his many little drawers.

The oldest brother, Max, was an oil painter. His most memorable works featured cockatoos and jungle scenes. I always stayed away from Max, wary of his continual bad moods.

Sol and mother went out in the evenings, and most of the time they had to take me along. I vividly remember the Brite Spot bar in La Cresenta, California, on the south side of Foothill Boulevard. Sol, mother and I spent many nights there. I remember sleeping in the car, and if I had to go to the bathroom I would walk in the bar and use their restroom near the ski ball machine. I really didn't like those nights; there were too many of them.

Mother and Sol were now in a relationship and I was part of it.

Even today nearly 70 years later, I still recall numerous occasions when mother would dress up and put a gardenia in her hair for the night. This surprised me since until then I had only seen her in a white uniform. I felt glad to see mother happy, always beautiful in my eyes.

Throughout the later years when I occasionally saw mother, she usually wore a black skirt, wedgies and a white or black blouse. She usually either smelled like a gardenia or Jergens® Crema.

This turn of events failed to surprise father. He wrote to mother and said she should sell Mount Gleason if she wished and do what was best for her. He promptly followed up with a letter enclosed with a power of attorney. The letter was dated January 17, 1944. Upon returning to life as a single woman, she was free to do as she pleased with what my parents had owned when married.

Today, I still have the letters that father wrote to her during the war. Reading them makes me sad. Upon getting divorced, mother sold Mount Gleason. Yet mother either refused to or perhaps neglected to repay my paternal grandfather, Doctor Isadore Rosslyn, the money that he had given mother and father to buy the sanitarium. Instead, she and Sol used the funds derived from the sale of the facility to try several business ventures.

One was a banana stand on Victory Boulevard in Burbank, California, purchased along with Bernie and Gene Gelson. One time I ate too many bananas and got sick as a result, avoiding that food to this day. I often enjoyed riding to the Los Angeles Central Market when they purchased fruits and vegetables. I always became scared when riding in the back of the big green truck with tall gates, especially on one particularly windy day when the gates rattled loudly.

Boosted financially by the success of these initial ventures, my mother, her boyfriend and the two brothers expanded the banana stand into the lucrative Victory Market.

Soon ready to move onward into other business ventures, mother and Sol sold their interest to Bernie and Gene Gelson, who gradually expanded the increasingly prosperous enterprise—which eventually became the statewide Gelson Market. More than 60 years later today, the chain is described as "one of the nation's premiere supermarket chains." Sixteen outlets operate in numerous highly populated and notable Southern California communities including Hollywood, West Hollywood, Pacific Palisades, Century City and Santa Barbara.

Today, I have no bitterness whatsoever that mother sold out her substantial holdings in what undoubtedly would have meant a significant sum. Like each of my parents, I've always been a motivated person eager to launch and manage successful business ventures with the help of other carefully chosen professionals.

Anyway, back then another business venture involved importing souvenirs from Mexico and subsequently selling that merchandise in the front yard of our little rented Burbank house on Victory Boulevard. On weekends people would stop and buy everything from feathered pictures, bandoleers from the bullfights, leather items, maracas, alligator purses and other odd items.

Sol eventually imported bananas directly from Mexico to sell in our front yard. The Mexican driver would arrive in the big banana trucks late at night, parking in the back yard with the vehicle's bright lights shining high toward the pepper trees. Working seemingly non-stop on an almost a 24-hour basis, they often would unload and leave before sunrise.

My mother prohibited me from going near the back yard, proclaiming that the banana stocks had black widows, which she feared. Signaling her love, she always checked my shoes for the spiders before allowing me to put them on.

The Mexico trips were paradoxically scary and exciting. We either stayed at the Caesar Hotel in Tijuana or a hotel in Rosarita Beach. I often drank Coke® from a glass filled with maraschino cherries. Whenever sleepy I would lie down in the curved red leather booth. Our room would overlook the outside, up a staircase with a long veranda. The windows of the hotel and rooms overlooked the beach, where I wished that I could ride a horse like other people were doing.

Most of the time mother and Sol would invariably go to the Aqua Caliente Racetrack or the bullfights, and whenever those excursions happened mother ordered me to stay alone in the hotel room. I often watched the Caesar Hotel waiters make the salad dressing. Especially upon seeing raw eggs get mixed in I always became perplexed at the notion that people would actually eat that salad. I later learned that the Caesar Hotel had invented the unique dressing.

An Italian immigrant, Caesar Cardini, an American restaurateur and chef that owned the hotel had created the famed dressing, which remains popular worldwide. Cardini died at age 60 in 1956. Owned today by the T. Marzetti specialty salad dressing company, the product is sold worldwide under a dozen recipes.

During those early years I had nothing to do whenever mother and Sol left me alone in our hotel room. Although TVs had been invented then, they still weren't mass produced. The room lacked entertainment, not even a radio, and so I ventured out. Upon closing the door I lacked any idea of how I was to get back inside. Wandering around the lobby soon became boring.

Was I brave enough to venture outside? Sure I was, going ever so slowly down the street as fear gradually overcame me. A couple people tried to talk to me but I just skedaddled back to the safety of the hotel.

Finding the right room became an issue since I lacked any notion of the numbering of doors. Upset and increasingly frightened, I sat alone in the Second Floor hallway until Sol and mother returned home late, my body exhausted and a nagging hunger gnawing at my empty stomach. Needless to say, I never did that again.

Happiness always engulfed my spirit whenever Grandmother Allie visited, eliminating any need for me to stay alone in a boring hotel room. I disliked Tijuana and Mexico, always dirty and never feeling safe.

My times with grandmother in Hollywood emerged as the best years of my life. She served as an inspirational light of fire while always powering me forward. We often went on long bus rides all over Southern California. Over time we visited almost all of the significant landmarks, enjoyed attending movies on Hollywood Boulevard, and liked eating yummy food at Clifton Cafeteria on Vine Street. Our other favorite food or entertainment venues that we often frequented included Hugo's Hot Dogs on La Brea, the Farmer's Market, Easter at the Hollywood Bowl and so much more.

Grandmother lived in Hollywood until her death in 1963.

Sol and mother continued spending all of the funds from the sale of Mount Gleason. They tried importing pottery from I don't know where. They sold birds and the pottery via mail order advertisements. By this time Sol had rented us a very small house at 1023 10th Street in Manhattan Beach south of Los Angeles. There, mother had me enrolled in Center Street Grammar School, probably about the fourth or fifth grade.

By this point life seemed boring compared to the previous years of our many trips to Tijuana. Now, I was riding a bike to school, playing sports but not easily making friends. I felt out of place, alien and unsure of how to dress. I wore jeans under skirts that I had to wear most of my three or four years there. I got snared into lots of schoolyard fights throughout that traumatic period.

Soon afterward, I got lucky enough to develop a cherished friendship that I still maintain today. Rita Mae Doak and I fell into puppy love with our surfer boyfriends. We girls would spend most of our time on the beach, watching them surf rain or shine. Rita's boyfriend, Dewey Weber, ended up with a large business producing surfboards. He became widely known, thanks largely due to his steadily increasing popularity when competing in various surfing competitions.

Rita and I attended Dewey's funeral more than 40 years later in 1993. A native of Denver, Colorado, he died of heart failure on January 6, 1993, at age 54. He had first gained fame as the national yo-yo champion and also a widely heralded wrestling champ featured in numerous big-budget Hollywood movies.

About three years before we met Dewey, at age 8 he had won the part of Buster Brown, a popular comic book character created by a shoe company with the same name. Now a few decades after his death, Dewey still remains so popular that numerous Websites are dedicated in his honor. A popular Website—DeweyWeber. com—sells a huge variety of surfer gear.

My former boyfriend, Gary Stever, an avid surfer, became a contractor who lives in Hawaii.

Rita and I visit each other often, both respecting our close friendship of more than 60 years.

Mother and Sol's mail order-bird business surged. We had birds stocked everywhere in cardboard boxes. For windows we used wire affixed to the material via staples. The big macaws liked the tops of doors, the creatures so big that larger boxes were needed for them. Mother allowed these birds to leave the containers in rotations for exercise. Needless to say, the birds naturally did their best to mess up our doors.

Meantime, my mother's drinking tragically had become too much for Sol, who came home less frequently. I also had become confused, especially when abused by mother amid her continual drinking binges. Whenever sober, mother shined bright as the smartest, kindest person in the world. Sadly, however, by 11 o'clock in the morning on most days she started drinking sherry. Returning home from school became a nightmare for me most days, opening the door to our Manhattan Beach home to enter a world that I can best describe as "never-ending nightmares."

On one particularly harrowing night mother awakened me sometime shortly after midnight. Bossy and cruel, she ordered me to sew little buttons on a large square of cloth. Her unbending and micro-managing rules required me to affix the buttons "just right," in a certain way that, all these many years later, still makes little sense to me. Invariably, doing my best to obey her illogical, strident commands, I was forced to wrap the thread of each sewn button at least three or four times. This effort to secure the buttons in a way that pleased her kept me awake until nearly 4 o'clock in the morning on a school night.

That harrowing experience emerged as just one example of her crazy, childish, overbearing, and unpredictably warped behavior.

Delving into a much-needed survival mode, I occasionally began sleeping between the box springs and the mattress—hoping she would think that I had gone out the window. Desperate to separate myself from her increasingly bizarre and continual abuse, I often scurried through the window before promptly slithering into our parked car where I slept for the night, sometimes shivering into the cool, damp air. Striving to rest and to attend school became a formidable struggle.

Mother's increasingly demented behavior finally became so violent that one night, suffering from a bleeding nose and blackened eye inflicted by her—literally afraid for my life—I bolted to the home of a friend's mother. There, wearing pajamas, in tears and terrified, I trembled while using the woman's phone to call my father.

To this day, I fail to recall the exact words that I uttered. Maybe I simply gave him the cold, hard facts about what occurred—how mother had lashed out violently at me, although I dearly loved her, doing my best to be a good girl.

Father and my grandfather Doc picked me up the next day.

Up to this time I had spent only a few miserable weekends with my father and his new wife, already having learned first-hand that she disliked me. My move into their home marked the beginning of a sad period of living with them full-time, while also going through the difficult transition of transferring to a new school.

By this point, my father, Edward Rosslyn, had become a practicing attorney at 8272 West Sunset Boulevard in West Hollywood. I remained miserable although we would go to the widely acclaimed Greenblatt's Deli, still in operation today on Sunset Boulevard, plus Edna Earle's Fog Cutter Restaurant on La Brea.

At least from my perspective, my stepmother, Averil Hurd Rosslyn, remained very aloof, an exceedingly attractive woman blessed with dark wavy hair that would have made many movie starlets envious, and deep brown chestnut eyes that may very well have ignited a sense of mystery—at least as seen from the eyes of curious men, all envious of my father. Yet I experienced a side of this woman that everyone but she and I apparently failed to notice, namely her aloof demeanor that continually strived to keep me in my supposed place as a mere insect. Or, maybe she was basically a good woman who never happened to like me. Or, perhaps her unique personality was incapable of empathizing or bonding with anyone other than her current husband, my father.

Despite the coolness of our relationship, I felt sad—mainly for my grieving father—when she suffered a cruel, slow and exceedingly painful death from intestinal cancer shortly before my high school graduation.

Looking back today, I realize that my biological parents were identical to each other psychologically, spiritually and in an intellectual sense—while also as different from each other as the earth is to its own moon.

Certainly neither of them could have possibly known that one day their tomboy daughter would suffer from life-threatening cancer long after each of them had passed from this earth. Neither could have realized the valuable lessons that each of them taught me. Collectively and individually, my parents helped instill within me the perseverance and a refuse-to-lose attitude that would eventually supercharge my own battle to remain alive—all amid my dogged, "refuse-to-lose" quest for answers regarding my cancer while in my early 70s.

By all outward appearances, each of my parents were courageous, always striving to open new doors revealing the positive possibilities that life can provide. Along the way, as almost all of us experience to at least some degree throughout our own individual lives, each experienced his or her own sense of intermittent dismal failures, and also enjoying occasional resounding successes.

Like my late Grandfather Isadore "Doc" Rosslyn, my mother and father each possessed an innate, hard-driving desire to ask difficult and in-depth queries whenever faced with pressing, life-altering issues. To her credit, thanks largely to these very attributes within herself, mother later was able to make valiant, admirable attempts to address her debilitating alcohol problem—determined to put her life back on track.

Surely just about everyone on this earth has within us, deep within our hearts and souls, the seeds of potentially boundless curiosity. Used properly, such attributes can work wonders, creating a pathway for the betterment of our lives—in addition to enabling us to overcome sudden or lifelong hardships. Little did I know as a child that one of my most formidable personal quests would eventually involve an urgent and passionate need to push hard for vital details, a life-and-death struggle to beat a deadly disease.

The warnings that my mother gave me during early childhood had planted within me the need to aggressively take charge when dealing with the medical industry. Ultimately, along with the can-do, take-charge attitudes of my maternal Grandmother Allie and my paternal Grandfather Isadore, all the adults in my immediate family permanently engulfed my heart, my spirit and soul with the gumption needed to persevere through the worst of times.

I suppose that whether or not they choose to admit this, the vast majority of people who live into middle-age and beyond have seen at least some of their relatives cry.

Certainly, I witnessed my biological parents weep separately in different situations. Yet this is not to imply for even a single second that either of them was mentally weak, or soft, or prone to resigning themselves to failure when the going got tough.

My own battle against cancer underscored the inescapable and universal fact that almost all of us are instilled with a deep inner sense of "right and wrong."

For me, during later life while deadly cancer faced me eye-to-eye, these pivotal questions would emerge. Primarily, would I be able to use the lessons that my relatives had taught, while also remaining fully cognizant and healthy enough to save myself?

Looking back from today's perspective, I can clearly see that the many events and life experiences that I endured as a 14-year-old and through subsequent decades instilled within me a fighting attitude necessary for survival.

Throughout my teens I remained a renegade tomboy who either had few rules, or refrained from adhering to any restrictions that might have been imposed on me. Nevertheless, a "good girl" all along in my heart and soul, while also eager to please my adoring father, I spent weekends using a mangle when ironing, also washing sheets and towels, and vacuuming—plus scrubbing a huge fireplace often used during lots of their countless parties.

Like many of his friends, my father enjoyed playing the piano and accordion. The widely acclaimed musicians at some of these all-night shindigs included the late Elmer Bernstein, who gained international fame and accolades for directing and composing many popular movie scores. His compositions for a seemingly endless stream of popular films included "Ghostbusters," "To

Kill a Mockingbird," "The Magnificent Seven," and "Thoroughly Modern Millie."

Yes, my father had developed a habit of hanging out with a steady, seemingly endless stream of big-name celebrities and various film industry luminaries, some of them lacking widespread recognition—while best known and respected by their associates throughout the business.

To this day, I know so much about my father that still makes me proud of him, not just his accomplishments as a widely respected attorney for many of these individuals. Most important, at least from my perspective as a teenager and later as a young adult, people seemed to gravitate to my father because he impressed them as genuine in almost every way. Rather than behave as if a typical, caricature of a classic "Hollywood phony," my father moved relatively unscathed, with ease throughout that maze of movie stars and film producers.

Just as important, father's actions spoke volumes. Never once did he sit me down to discuss or reveal the so-called "ins and outs" of the iconic film industry. Instead, his manly, gentlemanly and somewhat casual behavior conveyed to me a distinct message that Hollywood entailed far more than movie stars and making films.

Most important, from the example that father set for me I realized that he understood that Hollywood was more than merely screen tests, the film that goes through a projector, or the glamorous images of glitzy movie star lifestyles.

Above all else, he taught me that Hollywood reigned as a business about people—how they interact with each other, the devilish or angelic ways that they either cooperate or compete in a relentless quest for fame, fortune or world-renowned success.

Naturally, I became increasingly proud of my father, especially whenever photographs of him would appear off and on in newspapers and magazines, pictured beside his various famous clients.

Father's income increased thanks largely to his steadily growing and continually solidifying cadre of Hollywood luminaries.

This boost in clientele enabled him to accept two partners into his law practice, Bernie Lippman and Frank Schwartz. Gradually giving them increased responsibility, father seized this transition as an opportunity to cut back his court appearances, giving him more time to spend away from his busy office. He finally was able to pursue additional ventures.

Eager to achieve financial and business success, he decided to return to the sanitarium business. Naturally by this point father had become familiar with many sanitariums around Los Angeles. Lady Luck visited during this period, while I attended junior high, when he discovered that the Hillcrest was for sale. Along with his partner, local mortician George Greeley, father secured the lease and changed the facility's name to Pine Tree Lodge in order to help give the site a more pleasant aura.

First built as a hunting lodge, the property originally had been owned by a man heralded as "The Sugar King," John D. Spreckles. A South Carolina native born in 1853, eight years before the American Civil War erupted, Spreckles' entrepreneurial spirit had been instrumental in helping to build the early infrastructure of Southern California.

Well before playing a pivotal role in developing the transportation infrastructure and amassing massive real estate holdings in San Diego during the early 1900s, in the 1880s while in his 30s Spreckles energized the refinement of sugar cane in what then was the undisturbed tropical paradise called the "Kingdom of Hawaii."

Spreckles' massive holdings and business ventures, which remain legendary, included the launch of the Tribune Publishing Company, the original parent firm of the "San Diego Tribune" newspaper.

Surely my father's acquisition of Spreckles' former hunting lodge became a major personal victory, the makings of a potentially lucrative venture at a esteemed historical site created by an icon in California history.

Under my father's ownership, the lodge commanded

spectacular views for 180 degrees. The narrow and winding road leading to the facility had a gatekeeper to keep people in or out.

I later became surprised upon learning more about its rich history:

"Hillcrest Sanitarium, a large tubercular sanitarium located in La Crescenta at the top of Lowell Avenue had been commandeered by the government at the beginning of the war. It was used to treat the Japanese-American internees from all over the western states that had been diagnosed with T.B. Mrs. Nicholson spent much of her time with these dying patients."

The Nicholson Family's story is told in a currently out-of-print book from the '70s, "Valient Odyssey: Herbert Nicholson In and Out of America's Concentration Camps, by Weglyn and Mitson.

Mike Lawler, president of the Historical Society of
the Crescenta Valley

The book chronicles the life of Herbert Nicholson, a native of Rochester, New York, who became a Quaker missionary to Japan from 1922 until 1940, when he and his wife, the former Madeline Waterhouse returned to the United States. Following the outbreak of U.S. involvement in World War II in December 1941, Nicholson became instrumental in assisting Japanese-Americans as they prepared to be sent to concentration camps that the U.S. government had launched to house natives of Japan during the War.

According to an article by Nancy Matsumoto, Nicholson became instrumental in helping these innocent prisoners' obtain legal assistance and served as an interpreter during the war; he also helped transfer to them donated items including clothes. Using a borrowed truck, he made a "serious of extraordinary trips from camp to camp" across the entire country. Meantime his wife Madeline regularly visited Hillcrest Sanitarium during the war as the U.S. government used the building to detain Japanese-Americans who suffered from tuberculosis.

During my family's ownership of Hillcrest, the facility's large parking area always had plenty of space because only a handful of visitors ever came. Old and senile, most patients were unaware of everything that happened around them. Others were trying to recover from incurable lifelong ailments. For example, a young black boy had only stubs for arms and legs. He could only grunt when trying to jump around his barred bed. I always felt bad for him.

Close to my 14th birthday in July 1953, father decided that I should live and work at the sanitarium during summer breaks from school. So, I spent my summer vacation there at age 14. Many of father's days were spent at the facility. His other days were spent in his Hollywood office with his clients. While growing up I became very familiar with the property and all of its elements.

A small lake, actually a fish pond, near the lodge contained an island carpeted in bamboo and other plants. Only knee-high from the perspective of a tall adult, the pond was home to many kinds of goldfish—at least they all looked like such creatures to me. I often saw swishes of glittery gold float past as if watercolor ribbons.

The property featured trees of many varieties, including pine, green apple, apricot, peach, orange and lime. Everything was kept trim and neat at the stone and wood lodge, which had many rooms.

A kitchen below the first floor had an outside entrance. The facility's food-service staffers went upstairs to smoke outside more often than they should. I disliked the kitchen staff. Their troublesome behavior frequently kept my father in an angry state.

One day he walked in my room with something white folded along with as large ring of keys.

"What's that for?" I asked.

"It's summer. You're not in school, and I think it's time for you to learn the business."

My head spun.

"What will I be doing?" I remained unsure of whether to be excited or nervous.

Father told me that I would assist the head nurse where she needed me in Unit 1, away from Unit 2 where the TB patients lived. Brusquely, he handed me the necessary materials, turned on his heels and left the room. You didn't say "no" to my father, a West Hollywood attorney mainly for the entertainment industry.

A handsome gentleman often compared to the famed movie actor Spencer Tracy, he worked hard and played hard, too, in his Spanish-style, three-bedroom home on Primrose Avenue.

There were no ifs, ands or buts. I became determined to wet my feet in the healthcare field, in for the crazy ride.

During the summer of 1953 I saw too many sad and horrific sights. During that scorching time of year many patients needed treatment for dehydration. I ensured that everyone in Unit 1 got water several times daily. To keep the sane patients busy I showed 8-millimeter movies of anything that I could find. We made lanyards, key chains, dolls and anything else that I could think of. I played records for the patients and helped them with puzzles and crafts. On some occasions the nurses and orderlies helped with patients' baths times, which I detested. Panic erupted on one particularly hot summer day.

The county had sent a certain number of patients to our facility and paid for their care. One way or another, a huge conflict sprouted between the county and us. The government returned to pick up their patients as bureaucrats alleged that we had violated some of their regulations. Despite my father's continual attempts to rectify the issue, county employees conveyed a distinct message. They didn't care if the problems had resulted from their failures or ours. They demanded to pick up the patients on a specified, pre-set day and time.

I sensed something amiss upon my arrival at work that day while nurses scurried around, sweat cascading down their temples. These personnel pushed the patients in their rolling beds, and some nurses wheeled chairs outside the double doors while heading to the parking lot.

"What's going on?" Alarmed, I gently touched the arm of an older nurse whose wisps of gray hair were wildly escaping from her stiff starched cap.

"We were told to bring all the county patients out to the

parking lot. They need to have their belongings and records."

"That's strange. Why?"

"They need to be accounted for and moved to another facility." The nurse's nostrils flared with her labored breath. "Now, come lend us a hand, please."

Everyone hurried, very concerned about the patients' welfare. These people were mentally ill, sick, old, feeble, infirm, and didn't want to go outside during the midday summer heat of La Crescenta.

"No, no I don't' want to go!" One mentally ill patient shouted, bursting into tears.

"It will be okay." I soothed, actually unsure if his situation would improve. "I'll give you some water. Will that make you feel better?"

Other patients started crying, moaning and calling out names from their past.

The situation had become tragic, to say the least.

I managed to keep up with giving the patients cups of water, running around with a pitcher. But then that presented another problem when they started needing to urinate. The situation would have been comical if it weren't so dangerous. The sanitarium staff tried to comfort about 30 patients, some in wheelchairs and others on gurneys in the sweltering parking lot. The day seemed to drip by like our sweat, and I told the nurses of my concern that we would continue melting in the parking lot during this urgent situation.

After the number of dehydrated patients skyrocketed, my father's face turned to stone: "Take the patients inside."

He refused to let the county subject the patients to additional injury and stress. So back they went. By the time the county bureaucrats finally arrived my father was already poised to prepare a lawsuit against them for all the trouble caused to our patients and staff.

The county bureaucrats finally departed, leaving all of its patients in our care. This marked my first experience emphasizing the fact that health care is really a business just like almost any other money-making venture.

One morning a sanitarium staffer asked me to go to the switchboard, just off the main entry and near where all the office staff walked past. When I got there, the sun shined through the south-facing window, reflecting on the old switchboard and its cable cords. Unfamiliar with this, I became very leery of the task at hand.

Fletcher, the head nurse of average height had a nice figure and reddish, short, curly hair. She always wore a perfectly starched white uniform with her nurse cap.

"Okay, Diana—Grace will show you how this works." Fletcher turned to leave me with this machine and also in the hands of the other woman.

Cords and chrome popping out and hanging in an awkward array of confusion looked so foreign to me that I broke into a cold sweat.

Facing the switchboard, we momentarily looked at each other. Grace sensed my panic. As she started to explain, I began wondering why I had been chosen for this job away from our patients. I finally asked after politely waiting for her to finish. The regular girl apparently had failed to show up that morning.

Grace then gave me detailed instructions that promptly became a blur. She wrote the basics down upon seeing that I still looked vacant.

"You'll do just fine, dear."

With a pat on the shoulder, she left me alone. Having no one in my presence to personally answer to, I dreaded the first ring. I finally started to relax after the first couple hours of successfully completed calls—bad idea. As soon as you think you are clear and sailing, you're not.

I heard the creak of wheels out in the sterile white hallway with its dark wooden floors, followed by slow footsteps. Glancing at the doorway, I saw two orderlies wheel a gurney toward me.

"What's going o—" I abruptly quieted down upon seeing

someone on the gurney fully covered by a white, thick sheet. Nausea rose to my throat.

"This man has passed away," the orderly declared, as if this were a question. "The relatives have been notified very early this morning. They said they would send up a mortuary operator to pick up the body right away. We need you to keep an eye on him."

Queasiness continued. That was my job now, to work the switchboard and watch over the man's dead body until mortuary personnel arrived. At 14, I knew better than to reveal any weariness to my father. Failing to complete a task would displease him. With a gulp I turned my face away from the foreboding sheet covering the human-shaped lump.

Minutes trickled into hours. Soon the sun had long-since dimmed and twilight neared as the late-afternoon sunset retreated behind the hills.

Still no pick up, so I had no choice other than to remain with the covered body.

Wringing my hands together, I shuddered at the thought of being alone with a corpse that night. Finally, I heard my father's gruff voice while burying my head in my hands.

"Hey, Diana, go ahead and leave."

I lifted my head as he fiddled with the keys in the doorway.

"Diana, I called my partner's mortuary to come pick up this poor abandoned fellow."

We never heard from the relatives.

Many more depressing events occurred during that long summer, enabling me to gain two valuable insights. One, I could never be a nurse. Two, it's a wonder I didn't need therapy.

Chapter 2
Ever Changing

While a young adult, I gave birth to the new light of my life—Jamie Beardsley during the early 1960s in Encino, California.

Upon the subsequent shift of my family during the years after her birth, she became one of the most vital people in my life.

The other important person had been her father. Since Jamie's birth I've remained amazed by her generous and loving ways instilled by her father—a handsome, intelligent man. On the day of her birth, as parents we were young, unready for a child and for married life. Jim and I tried to make our marriage work but we were just too young and we had interference from my father. We were sad at the turn of events thrust upon us and did what we considered best for Jamie. We had been living in Woodland Hills, California. Now it was Jamie and I forging on. To this day I love Jim dearly and he remains an important part of our lives.

I wanted to rear Jamie in a rural area. Looking around, Agoura, California, seemed a very desire location. Rolling green hills and enormous oak trees covered the landscape, a virtual cornucopia of delight for the eyes. The Chumash Indian Tribe maintained villages around the area, rumored to have lingering spirits.

Agoura first gained fame a half century earlier in the 1920s when Paramount Studios used the region long before development as an ideal western film location.

In order to get a post office in their community during that decade residents needed to vote on a one-word name for the region. Historians insist that in 1927 voters selected the incorrect spelling of a name intended to honor Basque immigrant Pierre Agoure.

Much of the region remained relatively untouched by development by the time I initially scoured the community with Jamie. The region remained so isolated that residents waited until 1982 before incorporating the Agoura hills area into a city.

Using proceeds from the sale of our Woodland Hills home, I purchased three acres off Chesebro Road. Near the southern edge of the majestic Cheeseboro Palo-Comado Canyons. The road and the canyon had different yet similar spellings.

Our new property had been a pheasant farm, said to have supplied famed crooner and movie star Bing Crosby and his friends with fowl, built sometime in the 1930s.

Agoura remained very rural in the mid-'60s. We lived on an unpaved section of the road, our mailbox a quarter mile up the street from where pavement ended. Children rode horses and people raised chickens amid lots of gardens and fruit trees. Each home was unique, vastly different from the others. Some people had built new larger houses but the majority were old and small.

I felt happy with my decision, partly because the neighbors all behaved in a kind, friendly manner that helped make us feel at ease and fully accepted. While looking for additional properties I also visited car dealerships to find a suitable vehicle.

The fantastic property and an acceptable car each caught my fancy. Before long I started dating the auto dealership's manager. My relationship grew with Robert Warren, who had a son, Austin, just a few years younger than Jamie. Our children got along well and we decided to marry in Las Vegas in 1968.

At the time Jamie and I had been living in our rural "cabin" and now we had to make room for our new family. We managed this okay as Robert hired carpenters to complete various upgrades in the residence. Life went along very smoothly until my tumors appeared.

An internationally acclaimed physician still popular today, Doctor Edward O. Terino found non-cancerous fibrocystic tumors in my right breast from the results of a mammogram. We had been living in Agoura for about two years. I had been a stay-at-home housewife while Robert worked at a dealership in Santa Monica. Jamie kept busy with her activities while happy in school. Now I had to take care of this matter quickly.

Doctor Terino recommended that I undergo the simple removal of the little fatty bunches of grape-like tumors. After a few stitches in the armpit area I resumed normal activities within a couple of weeks. I never expected to find a friend during the ordeal. Doctor T's intelligence and kindness surprised me. His every smile radiated authenticity.

After a few stitches in the armpit area I resumed normal activities within a couple weeks. While I never expected to find a friend during the ordeal, Doctor T's intelligence and kindness surprised me.

Robert and I had begun living apart, seeing each other only on weekends. With the help of Robert's mother we had purchased a Pontiac-Fiat dealership in Manhattan Beach, my old home of many years. This meant him staying there during the week due to the long drive to Agoura.

Left alone, Jamie and I worked to take care of the property. We now had four horses and about 300 chickens, some cats and a stray dog. Jamie sold our eggs for about $3 per dozen, delivering them on a small Honda motorcycle. One scrawny hen with missing feathers would lay a new three-yolk egg about once a week.

Jamie spent some summers in Oregon with her father while I

remained busy. In my past I previously had worked summers with a couple of old contractors in the San Fernando Valley. My tomboy tendencies from childhood and youth carried over, my experience at that point formidable enough to attend contractors' school.

During that time I re-roofed our cabin, refinished most of the old interior and met many people in Agoura.

In 1977, I passed my General Contractors B-1 license test and built my first house on our second acre. Thirty-five years later in 2012 I finally stopped renewing my B-1 license.

When I had visited other doctors in the past they had treated me as a mere nuisance. Then he or she would scribble a prescription and all but shoo me out of the office. If I asked for an explanation, their minds were seemingly in the stratosphere, unable or unwilling to dip down to my level.

Doctor T took an opposite approach from his counterparts.

Pleasant and thorough, he always listened and answered my questions in an encouraging manner.

"How do I prevent more tumors?" I asked.

Although these benign growths had been diagnosed as harmless, this nerve-racking experience spiked my concern after learning of the need to watch for tumors to recur.

"Well," he always began, appearing to rummage through his mind for the right words. "The larger the breast size, the more tissue there is for the tumors to grow. You will have to have to watch your breasts for changes."

This concerned me because my bust was a 34D.

Doctor T always spoke in thoughtful, calculated terms. I hung on his every word.

Amid this period Doctor Terino and I went sailing on Lake Sherwood and socialized as couples with our respective partners at the time. We developed a friendship as I soon realized that this fun-loving doctor possessed a fantastic sense of humor.

Within a couple years, in around 1979 I noticed that more of those pesky grape-sized tumors had returned. From my home living with Jamie behind the Santa Monica Mountains, I rushed back to Doctor T in Westlake Village, California, telling him that I wanted the new lumps removed.

With greater urgency than before, this time we needed to discover the precise nature of the disease. I thought perhaps removing as much of the breast tissue as possible might make less of an area for tumors to grow. Then I verbalized my thoughts to Doctor T.

"That's a perfectly reasonable procedure," Doctor T said. "It's something you can think about after we remove the current ones."

I met my new friend Sharon Riddle in this idyllic neighborhood. She and her husband, Bob, had married right out of high school. Thanks largely to her brains and drive they owned and operated a heavy equipment rental business. We went on many adventures during our friendship.

We frequently lounged around the patio, propping our feet on the wood picnic table and watching the neighbors' horses wander around their field. One afternoon, Sharon brought out a current fashion magazine.

"Check out these styles." Sharon thrust a colorful page under my nose. "I feel like you have to be braless to wear clothes like these."

"Sharon, I don't know that that's something I'd be comfortable with." I looked down at the two peaks on my chest. She shot me a goofy look when we made eye contact.

Sharon's right breast was much smaller than her left, which led us to discuss the topic of bosom enhancement. We empathized perfectly with each other.

"Well, you know what I think, Diana—such a procedure would be okay for you."

I detected earnestness in Sharon's expressions, her face beaming at the idea of receiving her own corrective breast surgery. This led me to think about my own positive previous experiences with Doctor T.

Putting my hand up to signal that I had something important to say, I politely interrupted Sharon's daydreams: "There is somebody. Remember how I had mentioned my breast surgeries?"

"Yes, I do." Sharon's eyes focused on mine, her interest piqued.

Doctor T's genuine, handsome face resurfaced in my mind.

"My physician did it for me—Sharon, you'd love him! I trust him. You might as well pay him a visit just to check it out."

Meantime, I decided to have a breast reduction. My bosom would be smaller, but the implants would enable me to look and feel normal. The alternative would have failed to give me peace of mind.

After that day, we made our separate appointments to discuss our individual procedures with Doctor T.

Sharon decided to get an implant in one breast, and I would have a reduction with implants. Since we insisted upon having simultaneous surgeries, we felt very confident of ourselves—excited and nervous.

Our husbands dropped us off at the Westlake Hospital to be processed and to await the event. The doctor's staffers scheduled our surgeries for early the next morning. This gave us the entire evening to chat, worry, and hypothesize side-by-side in our shared room.

"We're going to awaken after surgery and feel as if hit by a truck" Sharon snickered, resting her cheek on her fist.

Lying across from her on my side atop the scratchy white sheets in our hospital patient room on the afternoon before our scheduled surgeries, I thought for a moment: "It's only 5 in the afternoon. We have plenty of hours to go! Why are we here!"

"Beats me." Sharon fiddled with her wristband. "You want to get out of here for awhile?"

The constant beeping of hospital equipment and announcements grated on our nerves—not to mention the anticipation that kept killing us.

My head nodded with approval: "Let's go to Cisco's," our favorite post-tennis destination. On many previous occasions their icy margaritas had cooled off our tensions and warmed our innards after rigorous matches. Soon after deciding to skedaddle temporarily from the hospital, our heads poked out the patient room doorway to survey the facility's bare hallway, and we tiptoed away.

"This is way too easy." Sharon whispered, nudging her finger into my arm as we snuck toward the exit doors. We stepped outside, flooded with sunlight and walked the two blocks. Cisco's close proximity to the hospital made our shenanigans easy. Over a plate of chips and salsa accompanied by one drink apiece we laughed and thought of our hilarious situation.

"To our new breasts," Sharon said, as we clanked our glasses together.

Sneaking back was not so easy. Everyone had become annoyed by our behavior.

"We were wondering where you were," said one nurse, her lips tightened into a horizontal line. We kept our thoughts to ourselves and tried to hide our smiles.

The next day after surgery we awakened to see Doctor T's smiling face greet us.

"I know you, Diana," he grinned. "I'm not surprised one bit."

The doctor had heard of our adventure, and assured me all was well with both of us.

My drowsy eyes closed, my body too drugged to smile.

At the time I had just began to divorce my car-dealer husband. He had been having an affair with a bit-part actress from a TV detective series, while his drinking increases substantially. I spent most of my time with a contractor friend whom I had met while he worked on my neighbor's house.

That's when I met Frank, an electrician that had helped me study for my test. I felt delighted and filled with a sense of fun when working with him, while also discovering my genuine enjoyment at working the business. The construction process energized me when laboring beside this man.

We built two Agoura houses, enjoyed fishing together and still had enough time to build an annex for the Agoura Animal Shelter at no cost to the county. Our tasty 6 o'clock breakfasts and the homey smell of the sawdust added to my sense of satisfying exhilaration during all construction phases—an enjoyable process in the '80s.

Perhaps largely due to our likeability and our mutual professionalism, we became friends with the building inspectors. The guys at the county's Building and Safety Department also were a pleasure to work with.

In the months that followed Frank and I continued a friendship with Doctor Terino and his then-wife Lisa. Frank worked on this physician's home and also the plastic surgery center. We enjoyed spending time with the couple for work or play.

Following my breast-reduction operation, my soon-to-be ex-husband arrived at the hospital in a new ¾-ton pickup truck to take me home. He wanted me to ride in this vehicle with my breasts in stitches and a drain in each one. The extremely painful first few hundred feet of this journey felt like riding in a stagecoach across a dry river bed. Finally, upon getting to the hospital driveway, I screamed "Stop!" and began crying.

"Please, I can't ride in this," I sobbed. "I'll wait for someone with a car to pick me up."

I called Frank, who soon arrived in my neighbor's Mercedes to pick me up. Finally, I could return home to the safety and comfort of my own bedroom and put on ice packs, necessary for a minimum of two weeks. I would have avoided the surgery if knowing beforehand about the horrific pain. Two tubes remained stuck in the breast throughout recovery. Blood and fluids needed to drain into small pie pan-sized plastic containers. The fun part entailed having to drain these contraptions twice daily.

My best friend Sharon's predicament prevented her from helping me. Thankfully, Frank came to the rescue. Smiling, he meticulously and gently changed the drains on schedule.

Contractors faced a difficult time finding construction loans when building in Agoura and the surrounding Malibu and Topanga areas. I had been fortunate to find a senior loan officer at the Los Angeles International Airport branch of Imperial Bank. Allan Blum impressed me as an exciting character who hailed from an exciting background. This banker had been a singing member of the Reedmen musical group, also a former clarinet player in one of the famed Tommy Dorsey bands.

Allan gained his own distinction by writing a classic and enduring song, "The Nearness of You." Historians credit the iconic Hoagy Carmichael for writing the song, the lyrics penned by Ned Washington. However, I fully believed Allan's tales of selling the song to Carmichael before it became world-famous in such hit films at the 1938 Paramount classic "Romance in the Dark."

Upon leaving the professional music Allan entered the business finance industry in Beverly Hills, at the time considered a Mecca for many of the world's wealthiest movie stars and families, plus high-paid corporate executives.

Still loaded with wild tales of his escapades as a ladies man by the time I met him, Allan diligently worked with me while carefully supervising my loan draws for various projects. One topic became securing a State Bank Charter from California's government for a location in Agoura. My intuition and logic told me that this presented a phenomenal opportunity thanks to extensive construction in a community that lacked a bank.

Three of us, Santa Monica attorney David La Faille, Allan Blum, and I received our bank charter in 1980, the year we opened the doors at Charter Pacific Bank.

Upon founding the bank in the early 1980s, I nominated for directorships several people that I knew and respected: Sharon Riddle; our veterinarian, Keith Berry; Gil Eisner; Barbara Dale; Pete Althouse; Ted Nehr; and Doctor Terino.

Meanwhile, I kept busy building a surgical center for Doctor Terino on Agoura Road. All our directors were approved, each becoming an eager learner.

Allan Blum did a good job serving as our president for several years. Doctor Terino eventually had to drop out due to scheduling conflicts stemming from a professional need to maintain his high-quality medical practice. Through the course of several years the board's membership steadily changed, a standard process most successful companies.

Several years after the bank launched, starting in the mid-1980s I became an "inside director," meaning that I worked at the institution. I enjoyed the significant responsibilities of inspecting real estate projects. My duties serving as Senior Vice President of Marketing expanded as our unique bank launched a new bankcard department.

Charter Pacific Bank was sold 23 years later in a $21 million cash deal to First Banks of America, also called First Bank and Trust. Three years earlier in 1998, I had resigned due to disagreements with the board regarding procedures and underwriting criteria. From there, I went to Heartland Card Services, finally deciding two years after taking that position to work on my own with special merchants. In continue in the industry today.

Chapter 3
Our First Nightmare

In the wake of a couple failed marriages on my part, since my divorce from Jim, Jamie and I have remained devoted to each other. As I said, she had gone through school with a stepfather devoted to liquor and lurid comments. So, the two of us left him, and we moved forward in order to leave the pain behind.

Fiercely loyal, Jamie and I hold each other when times get tough. My daughter had become a bit numb as a teenager but found inner peace although her biological father had stayed away from her during those years.

He has made up for those former shortcomings by subsequently becoming the best friend and loving father a girl could have. They still enjoy this special bond.

"He is who he is," she tells me. "I understand that."

I couldn't be prouder of who she has become. While kind and sensitive Jamie also displays extreme strength and courage. Never taking anything at face value, Jamie questions just about everything that can affect us. Happily packed with boundless energy, she flows with—rather than against—our universe in managing the smallest details.

Jamie's professional interests focus on voice-over, film and documentary projects. These tasks brought her to Hollywood, the Western Hemisphere's center for such opportunities. Since 2006 she has maintained a lovely apartment in a quiet, safe building. She often visits me in Las Vegas, frequently assisting with my projects when necessary.

While working with banks and card services, in 2005 I moved to that city because several of my largest clients live there, and others loved to visit the place famous at the time for the term "What happens in Las Vegas, stays in Las Vegas." Prior to this transition, I had spent far too much time in hotels, flying back and forth from California. I feel fortunate that when working with merchants my primary communications are via phone and emails.

Three years after my move to Las Vegas, in 2008 an accident occurred during one of Jamie's visits, drastically changing our lives for the next few years.

Amid this visit Jamie offered to take out the garbage to a huge trash container behind my condominium. Upon her return to my back door, I saw her ashen-gray face as she crossed her arms over her chest.

"What happened?" I asked, concerned by her sickened appearance.

"When I put the trash out in the dumpster I accidentally tossed out my keys with it. You know how deep that container is?"

"Sure do."

"It was empty. So, I couldn't get to my keys. So, I thought I'd get something to stand on and try that. I found an empty box nearby. I stood on it and made sure it would hold me. At first it seemed okay. I hung over, balanced on my stomach, my body half in, half out—but I still couldn't reach them! All of a sudden the box collapsed, and I fell back down to the ground. When I did, one side of my breast got caught on the edge of the dumpster, and I felt like it had torn my one breast off! The pain is excruciating."

I helped her to the couch, before seeing Jamie's tears of pain as she stumbled upstairs.

"Maybe if we get some ice on it that will help," I suggested. Walking to the Fridge, I grabbed a Ziploc® bag and placed it under the ice machine. Then Jamie held ice packs to her breasts all evening. An ugly sore, purple-blotched bruise appeared within a few days. Jamie cringed in extreme pain.

Many months later she still complained about soreness in her breast. She scheduled a mammogram back in Tarzana, California, to identify the problem.

Jamie later told me about the horrible experience at that examination. The nurse had walked in with a face of stone before telling my daughter: "There are some spots in your breast. That's a point of concern."

Upon hearing this Jamie felt like the world tumbled around her.

Later when describing that incident as we sat in my Las Vegas residence, she told me: "The nurse said this in a tone like the mammogram results had signaled the end of me."

Several hours after that examination, upon returning to her Hollywood home Jamie became concerned when discovering critical information on the Internet regarding the issue that her doctor had been concerned about. The Website said trauma often causes non-cancerous spots on breast tissue.

"Great," Jamie thought upon seeing this. "That's it—it's because of my injury."

Not so fast.

After Jamie's appointment the clinic recommended an MRI and another mammogram of the area. Jamie felt as if she were being used in an experiment. She endured these additional tests, probed and flattened amid endless waits in medical offices. The most serious examination involved a needle biopsy.

This meant the needles would be set in place for a minimum of two hours while medical technicians examined breast tissue. Following this continuous pain, a nurse sent the sample off to be tested. Days later, the woman called Jamie, telling her: "We're sorry to tell you it's positive for cancer on the side that's giving you trouble."

Jamie felt like someone had punched her stomach. The shock ran through her system as she responded on the phone, stammering: "Oh, okay. What now?"

The nurse coolly told Jamie to see another specialist for the next steps. As I later sat with my inconsolable daughter over a cup of untouched pomegranate green tea, Jamie ran her fingers through her long blonde hair. I placed my hand atop her restless one, her fingers strumming the tabletop near a cup.

"We will get this taken care of," I reassured. "One way or another, we will just see what these other doctors recommend."

Jamie just shook her head, "Maybe it's just because the nurse had become the bearer of bad news and spoke so indifferently. But there was something I disliked about her."

My daughter also wondered about the doctor that had been recommended to her, curious about whether she should open up her feelings but scared to death, briefly commenting to me: "Who knows what he's like."

Ultimately, as we would discover much later, Jamie had been right to have such misgivings about the specialist. Following that visit of several days to my Las Vegas home, Jamie returned to Hollywood to await the referral call. When the appointment day finally arrived, Jamie promised to call me the minute the doctor's office exam finished.

My phone finally rang just more than two hours after her appointment time. Jamie kept crying, breathlessly struggling to say what the doctor had told her.

"What is it?" I pleaded.

He had told her: "This is bad. We will need to take both breasts off."

"Both!" Jamie had instantly blurted. The news instantly tore her to pieces. I tried to calm her as she spoke, in order to understand all of what her doctor had relayed. Finally, she managed to tell me that the physician had explained details of what he described as the "necessary" plastic surgery.

He told her, "It's okay, we can build you two new ones!"

Jamie's tears and sobs at that point became unstoppable as this doctor declared while looking at her over his thick glasses, "We will need to do this right away. We don't have a moment to spare."

She went into complete mental shock. Processing cancer became one hurdle, while pondering a necessary major operation that needed to be done immediately exploded into a psychological mountain.

The doctor ushered Jamie into the lobby to schedule surgery the following week, soon adding as he stepped out: "And we believe that doing this so soon is by far the best course of action for you."

As soon as he left Jamie traced her eyes over the lobby where dozens of women sat with frightful expressions, many of them gripping tissues or mindlessly thumbing through the latest health magazines.

"Run for your lives," Jamie thought, soon snapping out of her dreamlike state when a nurse held out a card embossed with the scheduled date and time of the following week's procedure. Prior to the surgery, my daughter would need immediate blood work.

"We will see you then," said the receptionist, who promptly turned her attention as the phone emitted a shrill ring.

Feeling as if a zombie, Jamie shuffled to her car, her eyes fixated on the glint of the windshield. Still in shock, she knew the only way to make sense of her predicament was to call me. Naturally, I became equally shocked by this seemingly unbelievable—but true—development.

My mind tried to wrap around the possibility of my sweet only daughter getting trapped in this potentially deadly situation. My mind transitioned into a flight-or-fight mode, telling her: "Get out of there. Run away."

Within a few hours Jamie had returned to her apartment while still sobbing. We stayed on the phone trying to grasp her situation. I told her to call me after getting all the tests, pictures and MRI results. I explained that we had to get other opinions, starting with the doctor that had brought her into this world.

A treasure, Doctor Harold Melsheimer had since retired to the town of Tehachapi just north of Los Angeles. I planned to get his number or email the next morning. For the time being, I consoled Jamie while she cried on the phone. We needed to develop an action plan fast.

Doctor Melsheimer subsequently referred Jamie to an older OBGYN in Tarzana. Seeing him at the end of the week became a waste of time. She called me after leaving his office and we needed a new plan. Jamie made the brilliant suggestion of Doctor T.

Now why hadn't I thought of that? My daughter's cries subsided as the idea struck, and I nodded into the phone while telling her: "You remember Doctor T? I trust him with my life. I explained that this possibility had remained on my mind, hysterical and frantic since she had left the Tarzana women's clinic.

Lacking any history of lumps, she had never received a biopsy prior to and immediately after visiting any of these physicians. This situation was completely out of the blue. Taking all of her medical reports and health information, she drove to Doctor T's office the next day although only having a tentative appointment. The clinic's personnel had advised her to wait and see if he could see her. That was fine with Jamie.

She felt increasingly terrified while forced to endure the lengthy wait to determine whether she would soon come face-to-face with him. She felt so much better upon seeing his warm, friendly smile after so many years. He still deserved a well-maintained reputation as the best plastic surgeon around, highly skilled and knowledgeable in all issues involving breasts.

Following several minutes of reviewing Jamie's medical records, he looked straight into her eyes and said: "There is nothing in any of these reports that suggest you have tested positive for cancer! What are they talking about? Why would anyone suggest removing both of your breasts based on this information?"

Doctor T suggested that Jamie go see Dr. John D. Matrisciano for a breast biopsy to make sure. These physicians had earned mutual respect for one another while working on many patients together. Jamie and Doctor T soon became relieved upon agreeing to this plan.

Now Jamie's and my phone calls were about good news. Each of us kept wondering why those other doctors had pushed her to have an unneeded double plastic mastectomy. Is it for money? Mistakes?

"I just felt like they were money-hungry monsters," Jamie said. "They didn't seem to care how I felt about any of it, and they barely communicated with me…it's just like, 'Here you go, you have cancer. See you next week.'"

The rain cleared from Jamie's life at least for the time being. Conditions remained overcast, but sunny skies had thankfully emerged the moment Doctor T had arrived.

Meantime, a medical assistant from the original physician's monster-clinic made daily phone calls to my daughter, warning her: "It's dangerous to put this off."

The assistant persisted with these calls once or twice daily. In the process, this lady and her associates exposed themselves as imps, pulling on Jamie's sleeve to give in to the expensive, unnecessary procedure.

At this point we had known Doctor T for 37 years. Securing an appointment had been blissfully simple. The fact he had referred Jamie to Doctor Matrisciano never became a problem. Since Doctor T liked this man, we knew he must have been a competent fellow.

While waiting in Dr. Matrisciano's office, Jamie sensed that these patients appeared less scared, with a lower sense of urgency. The receptionist's sweet demeanor sharply contrasted the sour-faced personnel at the original doctor's office. Then there was this new doctor himself. His movements slow and gentle, this man walked as if among slumbering children.

Jamie became impressed by this man's attentiveness as he

spoke. His eyes never deviated from her except to scrawl notes.

"Jamie, the first thing I'd like to do is take some photos. Are you okay with that? The photos are to make sure we have many clear shots before we settle on a plan."

She nodded affirmatively and the doctor's face crinkled into a smile.

His personnel promptly performed the tests with gentleness and care. She stopped feeling as if a lab rat. She still had tough decisions ahead, although her iciness toward healthcare had started melting.

"Well, Jamie, there are two potential courses of action that I would like you consider. The first is whether to get a double-mastectomy as the other doctor recommends, or have me perform exploratory surgery. That's the only way to truly tell what's going on in there, exploring the tissue on that side just to make sure."

Jamie's stomach dropped as her heart, soul and mind realized that she would need to make a big decision. Both options mandated surgery. Jamie realized that Dr. Matrisciano would never know for sure whether she had cancer unless he performed the exploratory operation.

"It's up to you," he said. "It's your decision in the end."

Jamie didn't take this decision lightly. During a stretch of several days after this exam she frequently told me everything as we deliberated.

"I don't know if we should get the huge double-mastectomy done—I mean, maybe it would provide peace of mind. But this other surgery would make sure…"

After two weeks she remained up in the air about what to do. Jamie sunk further into her depressed state, each time the original doctor's office called about the double-mastectomy. Holding her hand, I vowed to support her under either choice.

Thankfully, over lunch with me she finally made the wiser decision.

"I trust Doctor Matrisciano." Jamie spoke slowly, rubbing her hand over her elbow. "I'd rather be sure before anything, so the exploratory surgery is my choice."

The monster clinic called minutes later. With each ring and subsequent gloom-and-doom voicemail, Jamie buried her face in her hand—plagued by second guesses.

Jamie remained frightened and terrified of pain until the biopsy surgery, worried that she may have made the wrong decision. I fulfilled my promise to stick by my daughter whatever decision she made. I vowed to say in California until she was out of danger and no longer frightened.

The day of the biopsy became emotional for both of us. I drove her to Thousand Oaks, arriving in time for the surgery at a beautiful north-facing building nestled on a hillside. Although both nervous we felt good about this procedure.

Prepping took a couple hours and once medical technicians finished inserting the needles we waited in a small room for Jamie's turn in the operating room. She smiled upon recognizing and saying "Hi" to Laura, a nurse that wheeled her into the surgery room. When teenagers these women had been friends while attending Agoura High School. I felt happy to see Jamie smile.

My heart started to beat again following the surgery about three hours later when Dr. Matrisciano found me and explained that "all is clear," no sign of cancer. Soon afterward I assured Jamie as she awakened that her breasts were clear of the disease.

Meantime the other clinic continued calling with superhuman persistence. By this point aware that a mastectomy would have been unnecessary, Jamie finally answered the phone with a vengeance.

She told them never to call again and that their clinic and doctor should be reported to authorities for the emotional pain and heartache inflicted upon her, while also striving to put her body in unnecessary danger. Needless to say, they had not expected her firm voice. I became speechless upon hearing my daughter give the original clinic these final words: "No cancer or problems were found. There was no bad tissue."

Looking back today, Jamie vividly remembers the explosive

64

emotions that erupted in her mind. At the time my daughter felt as though she had finally escaped being locked in the "Twilight Zone" for months. This bright, attractive and intuitive woman reeled at the thought that she might actually have gone ahead and willingly allowed that incompetent clinic to unnecessarily remove her breasts.

What the other doctors had diagnosed as requiring a double-mastectomy had been...

Nothing at all.

Chapter 4
My Turn Three years later

Las Vegas. Once you pass its city skyline—past the famous welcome sign, past the glitz and glow of its nightlife on the Strip—you'll see endless tracts of homes, apartments, and commercial buildings all in some shade of sand or cream. This city's new residents have difficulty discerning one corner from the other. The bland colors become boring amid many parks, schools, and normal neighborhoods. Mountains made up of low brush and rocks frame the desert or what's left of it near town. Some cactus and far-lying shrubs dot the landscape at the sun bakes overhead. In spite of that familiar picture of the place, many people from elsewhere initially fail to realize that the temperature plummets in winter, a dry-cold, with occasional stormy, gray days. A light snow—actually a slushy rain—can make everything outside clean and quiet around the residential neighborhoods.

On a particularly gloomy day of sleet I sat by Ken on our big soft leather chair. His eyes squinted shut while resting his whiskery face to the side of my right breast. I felt the vibrations of his purring as he snuggled me.

"You're very affectionate lately, Ken!" I patted his head and watched his tail slightly move with contentment. For as long as I had Ken he had always been a "tough guy," a furry loner who preferred exploring solo. I had never seen him so cuddly as on this particular day.

When the clock struck 9 at night, I gently moved Ken aside and stood, fastening my terry white robe for the chilly journey down the hardwood hallways. Ken slowly stretched and prowled behind me.

As Ken and I snuggled in our separate bed covers to get warm for the night, I wrapped my arms around myself. My hand slipped past my right breast.

"Ow!" I sharply inhaled. Glancing down, I gently moved my hand over my breast again. It still hurt to touch as I noticed something else—a tiny, hard, BB-sized mass.

Floodgates opened in my mind, opening a pathway for relentless fear and panic.

What does this mean?

Is this what I think?

How advanced is it?

And then, the kicker: What about insurance?

My HMO insurance at the time made getting an appointment a lengthy process, let alone the primary care doctor making a referral to another specialist. My logical mind and my senses accepted that the fact that I would have to call my Southern Nevada doctor right away the next morning. Understandably, I remained wide awake long before the office opened.

While still home that night staring at the ceiling at the tiny crack in the corner of my bedroom I realized that I couldn't sit and wait for something to happen.

Shuffling to my desk, still slightly shell-shocked, I moved aside files and documents to make room for my computer mouse. On the Google search bar I typed the obvious but still fresh and painful query "breast lumps." My fingers felt weighted as I moved from the "b" to the "l." Pausing, my eternally inquisitive mind truly wanted to know the search results. Each letter made my situation more real. I finally hit the "enter" button while squeezing my eyes shut.

The initial sites that appeared struck me as being rather vague and useless. Soon I saw a video featuring a Japanese nurse who impressed me as legitimate for a reason that eluded me.

Humm…

With a click I received the bluntly honest, much-needed information: "If you find a lump and it's painful, then the lump most likely is cancerous."

My mind dominated by intensifying anxiety and fear, I closed the Firefox browser and clutched my phone until the doctor's office opened. At 8 o'clock sharp, I made an appointment for 16 days later, the earliest possible appointment that the office could provide. Cognizant of the disturbing fact that each passing day would give that evil tumor more time to grow, how was I supposed to wait that long while maintaining any sense of sanity?

I ran errands that day to keep my mind occupied, such as visiting the grocery store. Typical friendly chatter among people struck my mind as mindless. I couldn't come out of myself, feeling as if a turtle stuck in its shell. Terrified thoughts dominated me. My father had died of cancer; and his sister, my Aunt June, died of breast cancer.

Getting over my father's death became difficult for me. Near the end of his active life, he suffered from a cancerous brain tumor that made him angry when causing him to start losing vision in the right eye. Never accustomed to depending on others, during retirement he had been teaching law at Ventura College. An avid surf fisherman, he loved being around the younger students.

A neighbor called me one evening after she had found father having difficulty walking near his home, unable to maintain balance. Concerned and eager to help, Frank and I immediately drove up from Agoura and took him to the hospital. Father kept insisting that a new medicine for a heart ailment had caused his symptoms. A doctor spent about 45 minutes with him before the physician came to speak with us.

The physician showed us an image of father's brain scan, a large growth clearly visible pushing on the brain. Within a few days dad's physicians had removed the large tumor. Soon afterward, to my dismay and sparking my concern we discovered while visiting dad that his personality had sadly transformed into a man I never knew.

The disease, perhaps coupled with symptoms generated by the operation, had hampered his brain functions. By now he viewed me as "young Diana," the little girl he had once cared for so dearly and lovingly. As Frank and I left the hospital that day, I unexpectedly erupted into tears, perplexed and fearing that I would never again encounter my father as he had been before wicked disease robbed him of his adorable, playful, manly, wise and strong personality.

Sadly, father's confusion continued until Frank and I attended his funeral just a month later. This once powerful, intelligent and great man left us without knowing who we were.

My family's difficult times continued when my father's sister discovered a cancerous lump in her breast at age 43. To her credit, my Aunt June had never taken any type of hormones, also avoiding alcohol and tobacco. Leading a healthy simple life, she had worked diligently as a homemaker for her son and husband.

When visiting Aunt June in the hospital I became shocked at her yellowish appearance. Her doctors had refrained from performing surgery, and no one explained to me what treatments she had been receiving—if any. A terrified expression engulfed June's face, her sad eyes continually tearing. She expressed her fears, yearning for any information that would help change her obvious fate. I left feeling empty, and her words still torment me today.

Although my father's second wife and I had never gotten along with each other very well, her death several decades before his passing had left another hole in my heart. Several years before stricken by cancer, my stepmother had ridden horses, raised Irish Setters, and became a super wife to my father. She painted rooms, retiled floors, gardened and cooked like a trained chef.

Around 1953 she began suffering from intestinal discomforts that refused to disappear, a cancerous blockage apparently remaining in her bowels. From that point forward she spent most of her time in bed after enduring a couple arduous surgeries.

My father moved her to Pintree Lodge (Hillcrest Sanitarium) to ensure the best possible 24-hour medical care, during the same summer that I lived and worked there. But her health remained precarious.

As that summer waned, father took her back home upon his realization that she likely would never get better at his sanitarium. For the next few years he dutifully cared for her on an almost continuous basis, striving as much as possible to administer morphine shots to minimize her relentless nerve-racking pain. Watching her body's gradual degradation tore him into gloomy emotional pieces that drove his heart and soul into a dark place. We all felt relieved when her agony finally ended. No one should suffer that much.

She is interred in a cemetery near the Burbank, California, airport, far from her relatives in Nyack, New York.

Needless, I knew perhaps better than anyone that family medical history makes a significant difference.

The two weeks dragged by as I sat in isolation. Unable to talk to anyone, I could hardly eat. How could I explain what was going on? I still lacked a diagnosis. But what I already knew seemed daunting. The last thing I needed would be for people to fuel my unease.

Finally, the red-circled date on my calendar arrived. I tried to turn off my mind. I drove to my lady doctor as if a broken robot. The nurse took my blood pressure and my temperature before weighing me. The doctor finally entered and examined both breasts. I explained that I had found a very painful, hard, small lump.

I lay on the table staring up at a seaside painting on the wall and wondering what such an image was doing there in the barren desert, before eventually asking the doctor what she thought about my lump.

"I tried doing my own research." I felt chilly and wanted to put my sky blue T-shirt back on. "I saw a video by a nurse saying that if a lump is sore, then the object is most likely cancerous."

The doctor pursed her lips: "I'm going to go ahead and say let's schedule a mammogram as soon as possible."

Uh-oh.

That's a basic beginning. But the designation ASAP means serious business, something that rarely happens in Las Vegas. From that point she remained silent while washing her hands in the examination room and eventually closing the door behind herself.

A disturbing thought dawned on me: "ASAP" was HMO—health maintenance organization insurance—terminology that meant "about three weeks." To the contrary, however, lumps of any kind must be tended to immediately. Still in the otherwise empty examination room that smelled of antiseptic and latex, I wondered how my survival was going to depend on these doctor's visits and insurance requirements.

Getting through each day became torturous. The lump in my breast grew daily at an alarming rate. I withdrew from everything and everyone, unable to eat, hold a conversation or concentrate on any task.

"What will happen to Jamie?" I thought.

Ken stared up at me, hoping I'd feed him.

"What will happen to Jamie?" I wondered again. She was my only family, her father living in Medford, Oregon, with his angry wife. I thought about how Jamie would want me healthy, to live as long as possible.

While pacing back and forth in the living room, I saw an 8-by-10, framed color photo of Jamie beside me. We were in Big Bear, standing side-by-side with huge grins plastered on our faces—raw, fresh, wind-whipped and tan. This photograph had captured our wild hair suspended in midair, ruffled by the wind, frozen in time.

My spiritual beliefs told me deep down in my heart what I truly already believed that "the essence of life, or specifically our souls" continue onward for the person who dies, except in the minds of those we leave behind.

Increasingly lonely, I tried again in vain to distract myself with television, yet relentless worries continued assaulting my mind.

I stood bare from the waste up, one breast on the cold mammogram machine—arm over my head, striving to avoid squirming or pushing the technician's cold, chapped hands away. I stared up at the woman's face—smooth but unsmiling while focusing on her job. She flattened my breast, moving my tender flesh around as if merely dough for the foreign instrument to continue gathering images. Unable to detect any alarm or assurance in this technician's facial expressions, I failed to ascertain any thoughts she might have had regarding my diagnosis. She remained stoic.

Afterward, she softly led me to a too-warm small room, telling me: "You can wait here while the doctor reviews the image." The technician then turned on her heels to leave. Left alone, I sat picking at my nails while in the uncomfortable heat of florescent lighting. Anticipation kept choking me as a lack of oxygen in the stifling room increased my discomfort. Breathing became impossible while my thoughts assaulted me: "What would Jamie do if I die?"

The technician returned 45 minutes later, saying: "Come with me to the ultrasound room." I followed, soon grateful for the darker atmosphere and cooler air. Within minutes I walked outside with the examination photos in hand.

My latest doctor had just recommended that I see a specialist—whom I'll call "Doctor W"—covered by my insurance. Medical office personnel scheduled that appointment for me nine days later.

Although I became increasingly angry, the evil in my breast had finally been acknowledged and verified. While walking back to my car I could feel the tumor, my heart becoming increasingly angry at what this disease meant—more doctors, more tests, more problems with insurance, and more grappling with the cloud of a potentially unpleasant death. I called Doctor W's office to verify my appointment, again more time, more waiting.

Shaking, I got in my car in the parking lot while striving to remain calm. I soon merged into late-afternoon, rush-hour Las Vegas traffic, increasingly frustrated and angry at the evil growing in my breast—plus the lack of people taking immediate action. The waiting became unbearable. Three weeks, then two weeks, then nine days.

As far as I was concerned, physicians at that very moment should have been in a rush to remove the tumor as soon as possible. I seethed. More waiting, no answers.

My discontent and distraught state permeated every activity. Jamie became the only person that I would see. She evolved into my beacon of light, giving me a view of potential hope in those dark days.

One evening while on my living room couch Ken sat beside me, nuzzling my right breast as before. This struck me as uncanny considering that was the effected side. Jamie's continual, relentless attention to my every need proved that she possessed enough energy for both of us. My daughter's long, slender figure appeared before me as she held a plate.

"You need energy and nutrients. Mother, you're going to eat something" She handed me an organic wrap filled with veggies and turkey. Unable to even consider refusing this offer, I appreciated and benefited from her firm yet pleasant demeanor.

Each night invariably became torture after Jamie powered me through those dark days. Wild dreams, exhaustion, staring into the dark and waiting for the sunrise emerged into all that I could rely on during those hours. My daytimes became just as restless, while nagging thoughts of my growing lump became all-consuming.

"This malicious thing keeps growing," I thought.

How was I supposed to sit still? I resolved to spend all my time on the Internet, searching for all the world's cancer cures and treatments. Maybe there were effective natural treatments. Name anything and I read about it and studied it. I feared eating or drinking just about anything, worried certain foods and beverages would contribute to the rapid growth that I easily detected.

The tumor had doubled in size during the previous weeks since that fateful night beside Ken—originally the size of a BB, now as big as a dime

I had become emotionally frantic by the time I saw Doctor W. While in the waiting room of his clinic, each laugh and the continual round of chatter grated on my nerves as if fingernails scratching along a blackboard. I felt ready to scream: "Someone please help me! This thing is killing me at the rate it's growing!"

Finally, the clinic's personnel summoned me to get my weight, blood pressure and temperature. When Doctor W entered he looked at my images and began asking a few questions. He spoke little and stared in the air, as if waiting for an answer to pop out of his mouth. This physician spoke of his concern about the implants being so close to the current tumor. Just 20 minutes after first meeting this doctor I got a distinct impression that he wanted to avoid touching me or my breast.

When I mentioned treatment possibilities he clicked his tongue and said, "Well, I just don't know…with that implant, it's difficult."

Too fearful to do much with my breast, he then sent me off to find a doctor that would do a biopsy. As I left Doctor W's drab, depressing office, I felt as if he had just removed me as though a blight, a mere annoyance to him. To that point various medical professionals had kept tossing me to someone else in this not-so-fun game of musical chairs—more of my precious time wasted while the relentless, invading wickedness within my body grew and spread.

Once again as an increasingly angry and confused woman I walked from Doctor W's clinic to my SUV. Medical exam films were all I had to show at this point more than eight weeks after first noticing the painful tumor. The wind blew against my vehicle as I sat alone I this physician's parking lot. The windstorm persisted and intensified while I mentally reviewed what the previous six weeks had accomplished: *absolutely nothing.*

A succession of physicians had either refused to or failed to give me that help that I so badly needed, particularly a specific diagnosis of what currently grew inside me.

I stopped crying, looked in my cell phone, and called the doctor that had done the biopsy on my daughter three years earlier in California.

"No harm in trying," I thought.

His nurse soon sensed my anxiety via telephone. I briefly explained my situation and asked for the first possible appointment.

"I'll wait in your office for a cancellation," I said urgently.

During this same call, I then waited for a long time on the phone until Doctor Matrisciano picked up. He promptly agreed to see me because his longtime and trusted "associate" had been Doctor T.

Relief!

The doctor's staff promptly scheduled an appointment for late the following afternoon, thanks to his promise to stay late at work that day to see me.

"Oh, my gosh! Thank you so much!"

My faith renewed, I returned home and packed, ready to sleep peacefully that night for the first time in weeks.

Chapter 5
The Battle Begins

"Hey, mother! How are you feeling?"

"Jamie! I'm on my way to California."

"What?"

"I have an appointment with Doctor Matrisciano at 2 o'clock tomorrow. I'll meet you at one of the motels near his office. Just pick one and let me know. I have no idea how long the appointment will take."

"Finally getting some answers, huh? How did you do this so fast?"

"I have to do something, all this waiting and wasting time will kill me."

Jamie became happy for me, eager to meet the next evening in Thousand Oaks, California.

(space)

As soon as my dear friend Teresa Cirby agreed to take care of my cats, I promptly made the last few necessary chores on the morning of my departure from Las Vegas. I hurriedly spread peanut butter and a lump of jelly on a couple slices of bread. I would need to drive straight through in order to arrive on time for my early afternoon appointment.

Along with the sandwich I put some bottled water in my travel bag and jumped into the SUV. I headed off for California on a clear early morning. Feeling positive, while leaving the Silver State I avoided worrying about the fact that my insurance would not cover medical services in the Golden State.

I wanted effective treatment rather than merely talk and worthless referrals.

The early morning sun served as a spotlight on my road to California, as if blessing the highway upon which I traveled. As the scenery became scarcer, I only saw endless stretches of brush, rock, and sand on either side of me while thoughts focused on my friends. I had only told my daughter and good friend Teresa what I was doing. No one else had heard from me during the previous eight weeks.

I became increasingly determined to preserve all my physical energy to survive this battle. Well-meaning friends had left messages, wanting to know how I was and what was happening. But I felt unable to even talk about my personal situation until after receiving definitive answers.

I briefly stopped to eat my sandwiches at the halfway point. My heart became lighter as my mind cleared. I failed to notice the fact that I had become unstable, unsure, off balance and angry. Yet by this point on the road I had started feeling liberated, lighter and tear-free.

A soothing, misty rain fell during the last 40 miles to Doctor M's office. Feeling relaxed, I had decided to avoid leaving California until all of my questions were answered and procedures completed. I prayed he would agree with me from the get-go.

Finally, in a sharp contrast from Nevada's brownish desert, the familiar vibrant, colorful trees and green hills reinforced my feelings of "being right." I became excited when turning into his parking lot. Once up in the waiting room on schedule at 1:45, I started shaking so badly that I could barely fill out the forms.

Clinic personnel took me to the examination room at 2:30 p.m.

At the nurse's suggestion, I summarily removed my T-shirt before waiting—mentally relaxed and appreciating this phase of the process for the first time. Then the sound of a knock on the door sent my heart racing.

A lovely sight following many days on my own, Dr. John Matrisciano impressed my eyes, mind and soul as being a tall, good-looking, gray haired, bright-eyed, and calm gentleman.

"Hi there, Diana," he smiled warmly, asking how Jamie was

doing before asking any other questions. "How have you felt about all that's happening?"

I had given his personnel records of my mammogram, the only results available from my recent Las Vegas doctors' office visits.

"Doctor, all I want is to get this evil out of my body. I can feel it; it's growing so fast. Can we take it out now?"

After reviewing the mammogram and asking me several questions, he looked at me seriously before he started to visibly think. We discussed the possibilities; we just needed a solution that would give me peace of mind. He momentarily left without a word. About ten minutes later the doctor reappeared with a young male that I soon learned Doctor M had been training.

This other physician said, "You are to go across the parking lot to the lab and get blood work. When you are finished, bring the results back, and we will get started."

As directed, I returned to his office 40 minutes later with the blood work report.

"Okay," Doctor M said. "We will prepare a room and remove the tumor now. We can work backwards."

At the time I failed to understand this remark meant; I would learn these specifics later in my adventure.

"Wow," I said, initially having difficulty believing that action was finally being taken. "That's great."

They gestured to follow as they led me into a small room, a white sheet covering a white examination bed, the main furniture. I also soon noticed a table upon which rested sharp, thin, metallic instruments for doctors to perform their surgical deeds. I lay down, and Doctor M administered a local anesthetic near my ribcage.

He bent over and cleaned the surgical area with an antibacterial wipe.

"So, tell me what's been going on with the doctors in Las Vegas, and all your disappointments with them."

While telling this doctor my story I felt he was actually engaged, truly caring about my experiences. His eyes crinkled kindly with smiles at my passionate retelling of my mind-crunching experiences. As he began the surgical procedure, my entire body, spirit and mind could have whooped for joy.

"It's all over," I thought, grinning. "This is what I've needed."

After removing the tumor, Doctor M showed me a jar of reddish-yellow liquid.

"Take a look at this fellow," he said.

If I didn't know better, my mind would have thought that there was a little hairy crab in there—a growth with claw-like protrusions.

"Is it cancerous?" I spoke softly.

"There's no way to know for sure until we send it to a lab." Doctor M placed the jar back on the table of surgical tools and laced his fingers together.

I nodded affirmatively, grateful for his systematic and meticulous approach.

I put my T-shirt back on after being bandaged, and went to the clinic's waiting room to make a payment. At this point I felt little pain or discomfort, speaking briefly with Doctor M about our mutual friend Doctor T.

With the messy job done, he spent time chatting with me about past friends, the surgical center, and why he wanted me to return the following week for a "clean-up" surgical procedure to ensure that the surrounding tissues and nodes remained clean. He also recommended that I undergo a usual MRI with dye to identify details within tissues. I could simply walk across the street to make the MRI appointment.

To my surprise, my legs felt like lead as I walked back to my car. My body felt dragged down, a warm, pulsating pain worsened at the surgical site.

I fumbled for my keys and unlocked the vehicle, unsure whether the growing, all-encompassing pain would force me to slump onto the steering wheel while attempting to drive to the motel where Jamie would be waiting. My mind felt a great sense of relief that the tumor had finally been removed. Yet these surgical aftershocks sent twinges of sharp, debilitating pain through my weary body.

"The cancer is out," I thought. "Everything will improve."

Intense traffic on U.S. Highway 101 in California prevented my daughter from arriving on time. But I became relieved upon seeing her smiling, sweet face. My wait in the motel lobby had been uncomfortable, barely able to move my right arm while sitting with only my car keys in hand. Jamie registered for us, got the room keys, took me to our room, and set me down with ice and pillows. Once we got settled, she went out to grab food and more ice packs. After an hour or so she returned with our luggage and food.

Me? I strived to remain motionless.

Thankfully, her attentiveness distracted me somewhat from the constant chatter and loud antics of construction workers outside, plus the searing breast pain. The increasingly intense, nerve-rattling discomfort became so bad that I almost forgot that I would need to wait to hear my fate, the results of tests on the tumor.

At first I only took half of a pain pill because dangerous and uncomfortable side effects can emerge. This temporary relief failed to last long. I soon realized that a whole pill would be necessary to extinguish the demonic fire sizzling within my chest. Nothing could be worse than being cooped up in a typically boring motel room, while waiting to learn the results of a surgery—except for the pain of the operation itself.

I noticed all the nuances of Jamie's demeanor as she tended to me. I often watched her delicate, sweet face strain as she struggled to maintain a positive attitude. Other moments she looked scared, sad and tired. Her clothes hung loose on her, already a size two at

5-feet 8-inches. I worried about how much my illness had affected her. She kept a watchful eye on me even as I slept. I'm sure.

I felt thankful to have a guardian angel in my daughter although sorry she had to cope with this just as much as I. Don't we all forget that our loved ones suffer alongside us?

The next seven days quickly passed until the second surgery, which had begun to worry me. The diagnosis of cancer failed to generate any surprise, although the type of disease specified generated concern. Although already feeling the hostility of this disease, I became shocked upon learning that medical tests confirmed its aggressiveness.

My head plummeted down to my chest upon hearing the news. Jamie became rigid, a petrified tree.

"It's Stage II and it's aggressive," the doctor said. "We need to nip it in the bud.."

But how could this be only a few weeks since its discovery?

Jamie asked for me, "What should we do?"

"She has three months at most to begin chemo and radiation once back in Las Vegas. And I recommend going back there because doing all this in California without insurance would be far too expensive."

The last sentence impressed me as sound; I had already spent several thousand dollars for the procedures thus far. Just before the second surgery on Halloween, he also explained that chemotherapy would make me bald by Christmas. This discouraging prognosis engulfed my spirit, mind and heart, which collectively and individually disliked the mere notion of such a horrific procedure.

By this point a new fear compartment had developed within my psyche.

What could be my plan for treatment?

The evil tumor's cells were very likely still striving to overwhelm and eventually kill my entire body, but I could control the path to take. However, another painful surgery about to get underway would engulf my short-term priorities.

At this point Doctor M's previous statement from a week earlier about "working backward" began making a little more sense. Soon I sat being prepared in the outpatient surgery center downstairs from Doctor M's office. Everyone showed kindness, as sweet as possible while trying to find some way this latest operation could be covered by insurance.

Doctor M held my hand as I lay on the table, telling me: "You're going to be okay. Don't worry. This is just important to ensure the surrounding tissues are clean. You won't be sewn up until the tissue samples and lymph nodes are tested for cancers…"

That's all I heard.

Then the darkness came.

"Hey, mother." Jamie's blonde head became a pixilated image that hadn't finished loading. "You're fully clean in the surrounding tissues and your lymph nodes are clean."

A general warm, happy feeling overtook me at this news before my eyes summarily closed again.

Tightly bandaged, I waited a day and then went to my daughter's Hollywood apartment to rest for the trip home. Drugged, I just remember a sense of peace and quiet, good food, and lots of love."

Two weeks later I finally felt healthy enough to drive back to Las Vegas. We made this a two-car trip because Jamie needed her vehicle. I suffered intermittent pain through much of that day, unable to take pills necessary for relief. I felt weary and overly tired, as if driving across country for five days, rather than merely the actual five-hour excursion of several hundred miles.

Whipping out my cell phone, I called Jamie: "I have to stop at the gas station—need ice. Lots of it."

Fogged from the pain, my mind subsequently remembered little else from that trip. I do recall the glorious end when the lights of Las Vegas flashed in the distance.

"Home and rest," I murmured with fondness. "I will plan my treatments tomorrow."

Chapter 6
No to Chemo

With every breath, those harrowing words from Doctor Matrisciano's voice echoed in my head:

"You will have three months at most to decide on a treatment: chemo or radiation."

I never believed in the programs that any doctors had presented to me. I would pursue chemo and radiation as directed, although I failed to see any logic in these deadly programs.

No one heard my cries for logic and sanity.

I lived on the Internet. I had no time to lose with only a mere few months to start a treatment plan. Doctor Matrisciano had no referrals for me in Nevada, so I looked up details on several Las Vegas cancer doctors. I sent him information about a couple of them, and he agreed either would be good.

Eventually, as a starting point I selected a highly acclaimed female oncologist. The most memorable part of her appearance became her lovely smile, beginning from the moment she walked in. Otherwise the appointment became straightforward and serious, as I had been rapidly lost weight. She began by explaining the program.

"So let me get this straight," I said. "Chemo is done according to a strict 'standard of care" and there is no deviation from them."

Her lips pursed as she nodded affirmatively.

I frowned.

With that nod, a new seed of fear sprouted in my heart. I'd read and studied enough to know for a fact that chemo kills both healthy and cancerous cells—rather than specifically targeting the body's organs with the disease. So, how could the widespread death of good, healthy cells help prevent a person from passing away?

Interrupting my heavy thoughts, she offered to take me on a tour of the chemo facility. Nodding slowly, I wondered what I would encounter. She turned the knob and gestured to the hallway, where I followed her to the chemotherapy room.

These larger chemo facilities were nearly always luxuriously decorated with leather chairs, expensive furniture and marble floors. I stifled a gasp as we passed the front desk. Shockingly, it had a bowl of candy. Thanks to my extensive research before this, I had learned that sugar feeds cancer.

Are they stupid or trying to keep people sick?

I glanced down at my feet as we traveled along, looking at the mosaic patterns on the floor.

My, my—they must make a lot of money. And they do.

My greatest shock came when we ventured inside the chemo room. Women looked up at me when I walked in. Most covered their heads with hats or scarves. Others were just bald and hatless, nonchalant when people saw their scalps. My eyes lingered on those who looked strikingly pale and thin as if at death's door. While poisons pumped through them, I saw their fragile skin, like gray tissue paper; barely able to detect the veins underneath.

I gulped.

The pretty doctor continued, tucking her glossy blonde hair behind her ear: "I understand it's daunting. We do offer counseling to help our patients accept what treatments should be done. It's something I would consider for you immediately."

She picked up on my horror, wanting to thwart the defiance that already spread within me.

By the third visit, I had become terrified of chemo, still losing weight and feeling weaker by the day. As before, I entered the waiting room filled with horror—more women, more heads in different stages of losing hair, no hair, and faces of sadness and gloom.

My heart and logic told me I could never become part of this herd of shrinking women and accept chemo in the "standard of care" format as presented. There had to be more. By this point cognizant of the fact that other significant scientific advantages had become available elsewhere, I refused to accept the "end-all" approach of chemo and radiation that this clinic offered.

My visits to this cancer center had already used up a month of my two-month deadline. I had found several other cancer centers in Nevada, Arizona and the Los Angeles area. I visited them where personnel were always kind and caring. However, none would deviate from the "standard of care" regarding chemo and radiation. Time continued running out.

My heart and mind remained desperate to find a solution that I could live with. But where could such a solution be found?

Maybe radiation was an answer. After all, a controlled dose that could kill cancer cells might work. I scoped out most of the radiation treatment doctors and centers in Las Vegas. Most had high ceilings and lavish furniture. Following visits to three initial facilities, I went to a clinic operated by "Doctor P" initially looked promising. Sighing, I decided to give this place a "go," hoping the facility would emerge as the best choice for my body.

I committed to six weeks of treatments at Doctor P's. After initially glancing around the luxurious, immaculate surroundings— walls covered in paintings and spotted with an occasional plant—I sunk back into the cool leather chair. Maybe I was supposed to be here. Maybe now I could rest my frenzied mind. Doctor P interviewed me during the first appointment and all seemed okay.

The agreed-upon schedule mandated that my second appointment would mark the start of a six-week radiation treatment regimen. Upon my arrival for the first treatment, I asked to talk to the doctor before that procedure began. An assistant promised that I could after being tattooed.

Clinic personnel took me to a separate room where a technician marked the area on my chest that would be radiated. So far, so good. Next, I lay on the gurney awaiting the radiation to emit from a very big machine. Before that process began, the doctor arrived after a few minutes and said, "You wanted to see me?"

I asked him about dosage.

Doctor P appeared puzzled while looking at me: "There can be no low dose, only the 'standard of care' accepted dosing."

My stomach fell.. I had previously been led to believe that this would be a pinpointed, controlled treatment. No harsh, widespread cell death for me.

Everything that I had heard and felt strengthened my growing sense that this place and its treatments were wrong. Suddenly, common sense and logic commanded me to leave the clinic as soon as possible. This new revelation from the doctor indicated to me that I was about to submit to a procedure that would force my body to become exposed to unnecessary risk and excessive danger.

Why would they treat certain types of hormonal cancer just one way? Why are all the doses the same by weight? An inescapable and undeniable fact remains, that radiation destroys what it radiates. This doctor and his personnel wanted me to endure many weeks of this invasive all-out cell destruction, knowing that such treatments destroy everything. Logically, why would anyone want to submit themselves to such destruction?

"I can't do this," I said, simply wrenching myself from the gurney. "I'm not going to do this rigid, narrow 'standard of care.' Excuse me, I just can't do this."

I left quickly, tattooed chest and all, stopping only momentarily to tell the receptionist, "Don't you know that the candy in that bowl is what feeds cancer?"

Her startled expression as the door closed behind me will stay in my head for a long time.

"Now what?" I asked myself. Fear welled up again as I resumed reading the Internet.

Following a recommendation received by phone from a Puerto Rican doctor, I had been taking Lifeone® for three weeks along with Carnivora and supplements. I had read about his treatments on the Web, but he lacked any specific information on my type of cancer. My weight loss continued, 20 pounds and counting. All my clothes started falling off me.

I sent for herbs, followed German protocols and researched treatments in Mexico and elsewhere. With Jamie's help, I juiced and ground up all kinds of pills so they could be easily swallowed. All the while, I searched for something that would kill the mother cancer cells racing through my veins. This disease enters the blood. I used every available moment to search for a preferable treatment.

I leaned my forehead on my hand while sitting back at the desk, and temporarily ignoring the medical bills.

My spirits and optimism perked up upon discovering that a specific test can show the percentage of cancer cells that "might be" in the blood. Although not to be relied upon as the sole source in making critical decisions on treatment, this test is still considered a general indicator of cancer cells in the blood. Maybe such an examination might emerge as my necessary starting point.

I flipped through my HMO booklet to find a doctor who can administer an Oncolab Amas Determination blood test.

The next phase of my journey took me to the Las Vegas office of an overly busy and somewhat abrupt foreign-born doctor. I flagged down a nurse in hopes of expediting the process.

"I have a couple of doctors," I explained. "I'm mainly here because the doctor who operates your clinic is close to where I live, and I just need the Amas blood test. I showed the nurse all the directions and the special box needed overnight the blood in dry ice. I carefully explained that the blood sample must be shipped in a cold condition, arriving at the examination facility within 24 hours.

This nurse's expressionless face looked at me: "I'm unfamiliar with that. What did you say this is?"

I told her she needed to copy the details of the instructions or the test would be unsuccessful. Off she went to copy.

Soon afterward, my two-minute meeting with the doctor went fine. She made no opposition of my request, and we had little to discuss thanks to my straightforward approach.

However, right after this the clinic's personnel were unable to find the copied instructions and the original.

Determined to get this vital packing and shipping of my blood sample on track, I then showed the doctor the box that had been beside me: "I could give you this and hope for the best?"

No, no. They vowed to find the copies.

Someone finally located them an hour later, but not the original documents. Frustrated and impatient while tapping my fingers on the arms of a chair, I told them that was fine and wanted to proceed with the agreed-upon process. At least at that point I could go next door to the lab.

I went there where a technician accepted the instructions and the box, before drawing a sample of my blood. Then, she left me in another area of the facility to pay for the test. While remitting my fee, I wondered with narrowed eyes whether I would be leaving my blood with competent hands.

"What exactly will you do with my blood?"

No one said anything until one of the personnel finally muttered: "Well, why don't you just wait for the tech to finish?

I shuffled the paperwork while realizing that my only choice was to see this through.

Thirty minutes later the technician reappeared asking me to explain the problem.

"Do you have the box and the instructions with you?" I asked, striving to stifle my anger.

"The box is in the back on the shelf."

"Well, then do you get the dry ice for shipping?"

She lacked any clue of what this meant after failing to read the instructions.

Despite all this confusion, the next day this clinic somehow managed to ship the blood, subsequently processed although delayed 24 hours and never properly cooled.

Several days later the test results arrived and showed "elevated component results." This confirmed one of my urgent concerns. The sloppy Las Vegas doctors had failed to properly package and ship my blood sample.

I shook my head while telling myself: "Well, that was a waste of time, money and blood!"

Increasingly determined, thanks only to my own tenacity after those physicians inadvertently revealed themselves as incompetent, I found another Southern Nevada lab where technicians knew how to chill and package the blood simple for shipping.

All along, my health insurance had been essentially worthless, unable to pay for these vital tests—only agreeing to cover the costs of the deadly 'standard of care' treatments that I had refused to take. The insurers' heartless, bureaucratic and mindless protocol in tandem with the dangerous procedures mandated by mainstream doctors left me on my own.

Even though I had found a lab familiar with the Amas procedure, capable of conducting the test properly, I found myself always needing to think two steps of the so-called medical professionals. More than ever I yearned to find a competent doctor, someone whom I could trust. Certainly somewhere there would be a qualified doctor willing and capable of deviating from the deadly standard of care etched in stone nationwide.

Chapter 7
The Godsend or What
Suzanne Somers Sent

American actor, businesswoman and author Suzanne Somers became my guiding light in her promotion of alternative cancer treatments. I hoped to find something worth gleaning from her books. Like Jamie, Somers had been misdiagnosed, incorrectly told she had cancer. Thinking that hers was operable, Somers had decided against chemotherapy.

From one of Somers' books, I made note of the competent doctors that she had communicated with, and then decided to call the physicians that impressed me as potentially promising. I called and wrote letters explaining my situation and time limitations. Interestingly, I got timely calls back from each of these doctor's offices. All were helpful and informative, while two moved high on my list.

Two doctors each offered low-dose "IPT chemo" designed to primarily target cancer while minimizing the anti-cancer drug's impact on health y cells. Both facilities send patients' blood samples out of the USA for atomic testing. I initially failed to understand everything entailed in this atomic testing process, but the basics made sense. The mainstream medical industry in the USA has never moved forward enough in the cancer arena.

Rather than get caught up in potentially confusing integral details at that point I simply focused on the task at hand. I dove in, sending the results of all my tests so far to both doctors.

"Here's hoping this is quick," I murmured.

My phone rang the very next day. Expecting nothing, I became surprised upon learning this was actually one of the doctors' offices. The clinic's personnel explained that they understood the time element and the potentially deadly results that might occur if failing to promptly undergo effective treatments.

The other doctor's office took nearly two weeks to call. His nurse apologized for the day, promising to take my case as soon as possible. I said, "not right now, perhaps later," having already made an appointment to visit internationally acclaimed integrative medical oncologist James W. Forsythe, M.D., H.M.D., at his Century Wellness and Cancer Treatment Center clinic in Reno, Nevada—450 miles north of Las Vegas.

I had become weakened and scared by this point, still somewhat frustrated following my previous fruitless, unproductive efforts with other doctors—who all had taken too long. At this point my strength had dwindled to an all-time low. My clothes size had plummeted from a six-seven to a baggy three.

Meantime, my loving and loyal cat Ken continued to nestle against my sore breast.

"Hey, there, Kenny," I cooed while he stared back up at me with his ethereal dark eyes. Petting him, I realized that he was fully aware something had gone wrong. That cat is a biter and a stray that dislikes being petted or handled. Ken's temporary transition from feisty to lovingly persistent made him increasingly adorable in my eyes, especially whenever he tried to sleep on or near me.

I had read about dogs and cats sensing illness and death, but never in my wildest dreams had envisioned myself becoming part of such a mysterious situation.

"Even Ken knows how bad my health has become," I told Jamie miserably as we sat huddled on the couch. "It's just so scary how long this has been going on."

Jamie wrapped an arm around my shoulder after gazing sympathetically at me: "All you can do is keep going. Keep writing, researching. You've done such a great job."

"I just hope it's leading me in the right direction. I hope this IPT doctor is it."

While squeezing my hand Jamie gave me a deep loving

look: "You're one of the smartest people I know; you question everything. You've tackled this problem and dove in head-first. Mother, you're like an unstoppable freight train."

My dear daughter kept me going no matter how destroyed I felt. So many tears, so many hugs together, not knowing where we would end up, but believing there were answers. Somewhere, somehow.

Freezing rain ruffled my hair as I stood waiting for my taxi at Reno-Tahoe International Airport. I strived to keep warm by crossing both arms inside my oversize jacket. I felt sick to my stomach and my nerves worsened the situation. Within minutes the cab driver's chatter grated on me as we zoomed to my destination. My thoughts refused to stray from my objective.

"I'm sorry," I said. "But I'm just not feeling well today."

He understood and delivered me to Doctor Forsythe's clinic with a smile. I gladly paid the driver and stepped out of the vehicle. A little snow remained on the ground. The brisk, cold air energized me, making my mind more alert, capable of excitement while also remembering that Halloween to January remained the brief window—the only period during which I could potentially benefit from a cure.

Is this the right treatment for me? Is this the right facility for my type of cancer?

Right away upon entering the Century Wellness Clinic & Cancer Treatment Center, I started thinking of this as a safe place. This facility felt "real" and homey although small, unlike the huge, typical 'standard of care' clinics that I had visited elsewhere. Homeopaths and other doctors of natural medicine usually have smaller offices than physicians at the large complexes that feature radiation machines.

Feeling more relaxed and less frightened than when I had visited other clinics, during my first visit to the lobby of Doctor Forsythe's clinic the sight of women holding lunch bags impressed me as a positive sign.

"This is my kind of clinic," I thought.

After I completed my paperwork, a sweet and chatty yet professional nurse invited me in to check my vital signs and weigh me. A staff-level doctor came in shortly and discussed some psychological topics about my past, my diet and if I previously had any major traumas and medical issues. After an hour, we agreed that I was mentally ready for a treatment program.

Next came Doctor Forsythe, the clinic's owner and primary physician. Calmly and gently we reviewed all my reports and tests, before he explained the IPT chemo process.

I told him that the only treatments that I had closed my mind to involved radiation and standard chemotherapy.

"I'm glad you haven't had them. It's very good that you haven't had any treatments before the IPT. That way it will be more effective."

Doctor Forsythe told me that many patients have received chemo or radiation, or a combination of both, before their initial visits to his clinic. He explained that those treatments make recovery much more difficult for them. Those procedures kill so many of the good cells that the person becomes unable to regain vital health.

Upon hearing this, I thought: "Well, that's something I've done right so far."

"Diana, what I recommend is that we send your blood to Greece for specific testing. Although expensive, this examination will tell you the exact type of treatment, supplements and drugs that can and will kill your type of cancer—while also ruling out certain types of drugs or treatments that ultimately emerge as ineffective."

Sadly, countless cancer patients worldwide and particularly in the United States endure deadly chemo every day—when, in fact, those procedures could never eradicate their particular type of cancer. In some instances the Greek blood test indicates that high-dose chemo is a patient's only viable option.

Any unnecessary administering of high-dose chemo could be prevented if U.S. doctors gave their cancer patients the option of a Greece blood test.

Yes, doctor, please! Hurry up and send it. Never mind the $3,000 cost, which now varies. This is my life, after all.

"Do you wish to continue?" he asked.

"Oh, yes, there's no question—I want to proceed as quickly as possible."

Progress! Doctor Forsythe's sensible explanation put me at ease. Finally, I had found a logical, deviation from the norm.

I felt elated during my taxi ride back to the airport to go home that afternoon. I felt an all-encompassing sense of relief, finally on the right path. In the process I had gained an understanding of my cancer, while working outside the "standard of care," now on a path to healing my withered body. On the airplane I leaned back in my seat, closing my eyes with a peaceful smile, grateful my blood sample was on its way to Greece.

The Greek Test

Within a week I returned to Doctor Forsythe's clinic, going over results of the Greek test and decided to start treatments. I became impressed when reviewing such detailed information.

Doctor Forsythe's clinic gave me a bag of supplements that would aid in the killing of my type of cancer cells. Here, I have included documentation of my test results in the back of this book so readers can get a clear view of what results look like for my particular type of cancer.

"R.G.C.C International GmbH is a leading company in analysis of circulating tumor cells as well as Cancer Stem Cells.

Through our high quality analysis at R.G.C.C. International GmbH, we are able to offer a full range of services to the R&D, clinical, and pharmaceutical industry.

By using the most advanced and innovative technologies of molecular and cellular biology, R.G.C.C. International GmbH manages to overcome some of (the) restrictions that are involved in the analysis of CTC's (Circulating Tumor Cells) and CSCs (Circulating Stem Cells).

--R.G.C.C. International GmbH, "Research Genetic Cancer Centre." Accessed March 18, 2013. http://www.ggcc-genlab.com

Once the findings of this miracle test arrived, I knew these results would serve as the light that would expose the weaknesses of my cancer's relentless killer cells. That day I excitedly began the recommended treatment regimen. At long last my gripping, insatiable fear went under my control.

When reading through the test report at the back of this book, you will see that my type of hormonal cancer could be killed by taking the items listed as generating the highest death percentages for my particular cancer cells. Page 3 of the report also listed the best supplements for eradicating my disease. Doctor Forsythe gave me the main ones right away: Super Artemisinin, Poly-MVA, C-statin, absorbic acid and Quercetin.

I read the last few items on the list, asking him "What about Immune plus, DCA, and fermented soy extract? I want to take all the supplements that give the highest percentage of causing cancer cell death."

He told me that almost every health food store sells fermented soy, but that DCA is not distributed or sold at retail stores in the United States.

Naturally, I yearned to learn as much as possible about DCA after first learning about this substance.

In the meantime, though, my IPT chemo remained important to think about. Some physicians and scientists view this process as dangerous, although doing nothing almost always results in death. When performed ideally as planned, the IPT process decreases blood sugar levels way down. Ideally, these levels decrease to the point where drinking one orange juice suddenly motivates the cancer cells to gobble up these sugars, devoured as the primary substance that the disease needs to thrive.

While feeding on sugars, the cancer cells open up their own vital receptors, thereby making themselves vulnerable to potential attack. Thanks to this biological process, at the ideal and precise time that the cancer cells rush into a feeding frenzy, Doctor Forsythe's highly trained and knowledgeable nursing personnel administer extremely low doses of chemo that specialize in killing cancer cells while at their most vulnerable. Miraculously, this process enables certain qualified patients such as me to receive treatment levels that minimize the unnecessary killing of the body's healthy cells.

As a result, Doctor Forsythe was able to effectively adhere to my refusal to endure extremely high-dose and potentially lethal levels of the most poisonous chemo. During the procedure, Doctor Forsythe's nurses would constantly monitor all my vital signs. I never felt in danger, nor did any of the doctor's other patients that I talked with.

I always felt good while undergoing three IPT chemo treatments per week over a multi-week period. After carefully following the protocol of these sessions, I left Reno while feeling validated with a new sense of profound hope.

Chapter 8
Supplements
The Soldiers of Battle

In a sharp contrast from my gloomy experiences at other oncology facilities, at Doctor Forsythe's clinic while undergoing low-dose IPT treatments I often laughed and had fun with other patients and his professional staff.

We shared our treasured Uli Mana—the only raw chocolate we could safely eat. Some people had trouble; these were the individuals who had previously been through full "standard of care" chemo and radiation treatments. Also, in some instances a certain percentage of patients discover from the Greek blood tests that standard, highly toxic chemo and radiation are deemed the best, most effective treatments for their particular cancer. The people who had received such a gloomy diagnosis suffered during and after those highly poisonous treatments.

Looking back today, the friends that stood out in my mind most prominently include a middle-aged married couple that had come for their third trip. At a different clinic the wife had gone through regular chemo, which had worsened her cancer. This woman's faithful husband had sat with her during these IV treatments, which could take more than three hours depending on the specific chemo drugs and the amounts administered.

This couple gave the other patients adorable and kind notes and little maps designating good, healthy restaurants, and interesting shops. This delightful man and woman remained devoted and kind to each other and to everyone else.

The husband and wife rarely chatted with each other in the treatment room, and just about everyone there remained fairly quiet as well. Yet the couple always remained helpful.

The woman tried hard to get well. Repairing the body after standard chemo treatments becomes an arduous task. Remember, as previously mentioned, our bodies react poorly to the ravages inflicted by standard chemo and radiation doses.

I sat near the couple during each of my IPT chemo sessions. While leaving after the woman's final treatment the couple softly told me that the wondered whether this would emerge as her final attempt at seeking an effective remedy.

The saddest story involved a man in his late fifties seeking help for lung cancer, following arduous chemo and radiation treatments at another clinic; those previous treatments had obliterated the bone in his right arm.

At Doctor Forsythe's facility, while undergoing subsequent treatments the man slept in a chair most of the time. Whenever awake the man always talked enthusiastically about fishing trips that he and his wife would take, and hoping to enjoy similar excursions again. They decided to sell their motor home because she was unable to drive the vehicle. Whenever failing to distract himself by discussing his hopeful future while awake, this man's wide-open eyes looked scared, seemingly bewildered by his current situation and also in denial about the loss of bone in his arm.

The wife said to me while her husband slept, nodding her approval: "I'm glad Doctor Forsythe is treating him logically and sanely."

The IV rooms at this clinic were nearly full most days. Luckily, I was one of only two patients who had IPT treatments without any radiation. Most patients there were trying to recover from "standard of care" treatments that they had received elsewhere.

"Did your doctors at other clinics try to scare you into getting the 'whole treatment?'" one patient asked me. "The weeks of too much chemo, too much radiation, they try to pressure you into taking?"

"Oh, yes," I nodded affirmatively. "They were so aggressive—insisting on personal counseling if we have qualms about the

100

'standard of care.'…That without it we couldn't survive!"

We both laughed bitterly.

Everyone had stories about doctors pushing treatments toward us in a businesslike manner. And if those physicians initially failed to convince us to take the poisonous route, they then proceeded to urgently and liberally employ scare tactics. Thankfully, the majority of patients at Doctor Forsythe's clinic had prevailed against those other doctors, thereby putting themselves on a potential road to recovery.

I had felt good during the first week of chemo, but during the second week digesting the supplements became increasingly difficult. My throat became raw by the end of my chemo.

Once home, I began my pill regimen, taking all of the recommended substances three times daily in strict accordance with Doctor Forsythe's instructions. All told, I took about 14 pills daily with a couple liquids.

Soy that I had purchased in powder form emerged as the worst. My stomach immediately fought back. My day always became ruined no matter how or when I ingested soy. I avoided any thought of seeing people or going out to eat during this period because my stomach had become far too volatile. Even so, despite the discomfort, I remained motivated to take soy, never seriously considering the option of stopping this substance, deemed a tremendous player in murdering villainous cancer cells.

Back to the Internet!

Gleaning critical information from Websites published worldwide, I discovered that DCA could easily be obtained via mail. Following several hours and nights of searching, I discovered that many scientists and patients believe that some of the best fermented soy is produced in China. I refused to let anything stop me from identifying and amassing a comprehensive list destined to individually and collectively become my cancer cell killers.

Nonetheless, my tired but highly motivated mind began wondering how long I could continue these essential efforts, amid continuous nagging stomach ailments and research challenges. Still head-strong and increasingly committed to regaining good health, my spirit and heart remained fully devoted to finding and taking the "best troops for my body." The alternative remained unthinkable with each passing day. So, I hurriedly pushed any negative thoughts from my mind.

My only sensible option became to withstand the pain and frustration, because continuing my quest had become necessary for my survival.

Upon the completion of my IPT treatments, I felt as if a military inductee leaving an intense, arduous boot camp.

The second week of chemo had gone well. I developed a knack for smashing the pills and mixing them with different substances.

"Now, where on earth can I get this Chinese mix of fermented soy?' I muttered, after discovering the ideal product for this, Haelan 951. My Las Vegas condo remained messy, bills lining the desk, along with a plethora of pill and supplement bottles. Still weak without growing stronger, I planted my tiny body in a swivel chair in front of the computer and continued my essential research.

For the Haelan 951, I decided on a place in Utah, primarily thanks to that distributor's close proximity to Las Vegas. Although I felt nervous when initially calling and talking with the fellows up there, they impressed me as pleasant and reassuring. Personnel at this retailer had been selling the fermented soy for some time and were eager to offer the critical information that I needed.

All retailers selling this product require about $50 per bottle. That set me back because without insurance support I already had been spending large sums in my focused and continual efforts to eradicate my dangerously high Stage II cancer. I knew what I had to do.

"I'll take it. Rush a half a case."

I cleared my throat while swallowing a pill after this phone call. My neck strained at the moment, radiating a warm, raw pain. This discomfort had steadily worsened during the previous several weeks, to the point where I lost any concept on how to continue choking down and swallowing more. Pondering this while awaiting the golden elixir, I suddenly recalled Doctor Forsythe saying that "Haelan 951 tastes so bad that I cannot get any patients to take it, even in the direst of circumstances."

This served as a strong indication to me that this must be good stuff, just awful tasting.

I read newsletters and books by Ty Bollinger, the author of numerous hot-selling anti-cancer books, amid my continuous Internet roaming. He proclaims as excellent a green tea product, "Coco Complete," once called "Coco Pure." I had been using this for a hot drink, on soy or sugarless almond ice cream, already happy with the product. I became hopeful that perhaps mixing Coco Complete in the soy liquid might solve the taste problem. I'd have to see what tasted right once my order arrived.

I continued losing weight while still feeling sickly and weak. The IPT treatments in Reno had been an improvement, but I remained exhausted. Thankfully, at night while on the couch I could simply turn my head 90 degrees and see Jamie's sunshiny face and feel her positive energy.

Months earlier upon tearfully learning of my cancer she had told me, "Mother, my life is on hold until you're better. I'm your full-time nurse."

I lacked anything to complain about as she faithfully remained my only family. The love and support between the two of us became powerful enough to give a 15-person family a run for their money.

"Mother, the Haelan is here," Jamie shouted from the kitchen phone as I rested against just one pillow while lying on the couch. I soon saw her willowy legs stride over to me. "I'm going now to pick it up at the UPS store."

"Thank goodness!" I said copiously as she grabbed the keys and walked out the door.

Jamie gently placed the box on the counter as soon as she returned. She grabbed scissors and ripped the box, swiftly extracting one bottle for me.

"You know," she said, gently swishing the liquid before smiling curiously and pouring half a glass in front of me. "I wonder how bad this could really be."

"I guess I'll find out."

I brought the glass to my lips and took a big swallow. My face crinkled involuntarily in on itself like a bulldog as I tried to suppress the nausea. Jamie frowned upon seeing my pained expression.

"So, mom, pretty bad, huh?"

"Ugh, yes! Horrible." I grabbed and chugged the nearest glass of water before nodding:

Although I have never tasted break fluid the tastes surely were similar.

I then poured the remaining Haelan into another glass, added the Coco Pure powder and stirred. That failed to mask the rotten flavor, but I managed to swallow anyway followed by lots of water. Now I understood why no one wanted to take this. Nonetheless, I remained determined to take Haelan often, so what could be added to make the taste palatable? I searched for healthy mixes what would avoid interfering with this essential product. Sugar, agave and honey remained on my list of forbidden options.

Jamie grabbed her jacket and started heading back out again, saying "Be right back, mother."

"We'll just try this again after I'm back—you'll see."

She returned bounding through the door about 30 minutes later. Jamie handed me a bag containing lots of little bottles rattling around. While taking them from the bag I felt delighted upon seeing these were all flavors to sweeten coffee and tea that all sounded promising—chocolate, chocolate raspberry, orange, root beer, coffee, vanilla crème, apricot, English toffee and peppermint.

Jamie explained that these were stevia drops produced from a sweet but non-sugar plant.

"I bought one of every flavor so that you could choose which one you like best."

"Smart girl."

From then on I began using Coco Pure and any one of the stevia flavors when taking my Haelan 951. I started drinking one-third of a bottle daily in the mornings, chased by a large glass of water.

My confidence surged with the taste problem conquered while continuing onward to investigate the mysterious DCA, known to eliminate tumors. Determined to prevent such growths from returning to my body, I initially became disappointed upon discovering that the Internet lacked vital information on how people could obtain and use this product.

I accidentally found a Website that described results regarding the use of DCA on an animal in the United Kingdom. A veterinarian had used the substance on a large dog that weighed more than 70 pounds. The dog's owner had given the veterinarian permission to administer DCA on the pet as tumors were killing the animal. There was nothing to lose.

The vet started administering low measurements of DCA to the dog, unsure of the optimal dosage. The veterinarian gradually increased the dosage, and after three weeks the pet showed slight improvements. The elated owners allowed the vet to continue. The dog's tumors disappeared within several weeks, as the dog gradually resumed wagging his tail and happily exploring.

"Okay, not bad," I said to myself.

I decided to order a bottle of DCA after again reviewing the list of substances deemed most effective at killing my cancer cells. What would arrive, capsules, pills or liquid? Lord knows that another pill was the last thing I wanted or needed.

My little package arrived in two weeks. Boosted by a slight health improvement, I felt delighted at being able to drive to the UPS store to get the delivery. Thankfully, the Haelan had enabled me to regain at least some of my strength to the point where driving and most normal activities became possible. Though still a bit shaky, I ripped open the package to find a bottle of fine, white powder.

This time I faced the challenging of determining my optimal doses of DCA, which only cost about $70. I asked many people including doctors, none of whom had any suggestions. Only a few Websites mentioned DCA, so I posed my query on an Internet chat room where cancer patients and people with relatives or friends suffering from the disease discuss how and what they feel along with their results.

I spent a few days reading all the chats, suggestions, reactions and general comments. Thanks to my tenacious persistence, I finally found a comment saying to start at five milligrams before adjusting from there. Unsure of exactly what to do, I thought, "Since the dog is alive, I'll try his dose."

I planned my daily doses using one-eighth of a teaspoon, mixed with caffeinated black tea, along with the suggested combination of one cap of Vitamin B1. I became excited to see if my blood test indicator known as a "tumor marker" would improve.

My initial experience went well for a couple of weeks as I took DCA daily along with the other meds and supplements. Within five days after initially taking Haelan I had been eating and sleeping well, occasionally venturing out for short excursions with Jamie.

Everything began changing when I began experiencing a slight occasional dizziness by the third week. Six weeks after starting the DCA I had to hold on to the walls to keep straight. Otherwise I would have been walking at a slant. I became too shaky to drive.

This discouraged me since prior to that point I had been feeling much better.

But now the fear returned. Remember, my father had died of a cancerous brain tumor in the '70s, so I felt worried that perhaps the disease had spread there in me as well. I strived to avoid thinking about this dreaded, terrifying possibility. My staggering had become so bad that I shakily dragged my finger down a list of local doctors under my insurance. All throughout this journey that greedy, heartless corporation would only pay for the poisonous, deadly "standard of care" treatments that I had managed to avoid. These companies instantly deny treatment outside of their rigid rules. I selected a young doctor that practiced medicine near my home.

"Hopefully, he will avoid mocking my decision for alternative treatment," I thought nervously. So far, many of my doctors had been hit or miss. I hoped this one would earn my trust.

When my appointment date came Doctor Swaine displayed a keen sense of understanding, and his face brightened with interest while I explained my previous refusal to follow the "standard of care."

"What should I do?" I asked.

"Knowing that your father passed away from a brain tumor, I suggest a brain scan and some vein tests," Doctor Swaine said, after carefully looking through his notes on my file.

A new department of terror opened in my heart as I agreed to the examination.

The brain scan took up some time and energy, but soon proved that only things that belonged in my skull were there. I discussed all the possibilities with Jamie as my need to hold onto walls persisted, still taking all the same meds and supplements.

I deliberated, eventually telling her, "I suppose that the most logical, effective course of action would be for me to systematically eliminate each from my medical regimen every few weeks—until, hopefully, we can positively identify the culprit.

Jamie suggested that I start with the most recent, DCA, and from that point progress to the various substances that I had added in phases.

As planned, we started eliminating potential suspects. Following Jamie's advice, I started with the DCA, deciding to avoid taking it for two weeks. Within days I regained my natural ability to walk down the hallways without leaning against walls.

I had overdosed on DCA.

No one on the chat sites had mentioned extreme dizziness as a reaction, only discussing headaches or other minor annoyances. I reached a conclusion that "everyone is different."

After waiting an additional week to fully eliminate this substance from my body, I decided to take only a small pinch of DCA twice weekly. My research had indicated that this substance never accumulates in the body. I finally stopped taking DCA one year after initially taking this product, deciding the regimen was no longer necessary after my tumor markers had decreased to 26, a relatively harmless level.

Chapter 9
Ken Stops Cuddling

Paradoxically, Jamie and I became both stunned and delighted when my hunger and ability to eat surprisingly returned. My health had clearly improved although my energy remained low. I initially failed to notice the change, busy trying to chop vegetables and fruits and eat in accordance with a typically healthy anti-cancer cancer diet.

One day Jamie grabbed a slice of apple and chewed with a jubilant gleam in her eyes, proclaiming: "Mother, you look much better! Not so gray and gaunt."

I had been making major progress since incorporating Haelan 951 into my routine. Prior to initially taking this and for a period afterward, various other supplements and foods had failed to boost my energy and overall health.

These various substances or foods that never generated sufficient improvements other than detoxifying results in certain instances had included: a list of supplements provided by a Puerto Rican doctor; LifeOne™; Iiodoral™, a high-potency supplement; immunity-boosting substances including mushrooms, IimmPower™ veggie capsules, Carnivor™; Pau D'Arco tea, and numerous other substances.

The IPT chemo had broken off some of my hair, which finally started growing again, surprisingly curly. The hair growth started three months after I began taking three Biotin Forte doses daily—not just biotin, which lacks the full desired effectiveness when taken alone.

Meantime, Doctor Forsythe had sent me to Doctor Milne in Las Vegas to continue IV support and for monthly visits to maintain natural hormone balance. The average cancer patient's tumor marker can be 38; mine had now dipped to 21. To that point I had not visited California since my two surgeries. I regularly fax Doctor Matrisciano results of my blood tests to show him my progress, which keeps improving.

Ken gradually stopped sleeping nestled against my right breast. He resumed his life as a cat on the prowl. This transition served as my final indicator of success, my perceptive stray returning to his old tricks.

Jamie still considered her journeys to my mailbox a great adventure, delighted and intrigued upon regularly discovering something new had come. My body agreeably ingested and benefited from many of these arrivals, while rejecting others. Thankfully, I had Jamie around to remind me to take everything on time on a regular basis.

She frequently emphasized this as "very important."

Believe me, I knew.

My healing continues to this day.

As my strength and good health returned, I realized just how much the "standard of care" and rules that traditional oncologists must follow are preventing people from getting potentially effective treatments and getting well.

Amid my struggles I discovered to my great disappointment that the standard, cookie-cutter mainstream medical industry uses a truly one-size-fits-all approach. To the great detriment of our American society, this happens regardless of every patient's particular type of cancer and the varying sizes and progressions of tumors. From the view of such doctors there is and never should be any room for discussion on natural remedies that have helped me another patients, proven in other countries as effective, non-toxic, non-poisonous treatments.

Cancer hits at least one out of every five Americans at some point during their lifetime. Many people have called to ask me how I have regained good health.

One of my primary goals in life has become informing people that effective non-toxic remedies are available for many people with cancer. When time, resources and opportunity permit many cancer patients can avoid the poisonous and dangerous treatments mandated by the mainstream medical industry.

I strongly suggest to every person recently diagnosed with cancer to get separate opinions from at least two or three doctors—preferably including at least one qualified physician licensed to administer natural, non-toxic treatments. For Jamie and I, this eventual discovery made our arduous journey worthwhile.

In the 1980s my gynecologist had given me a prescription of conjugated estrogen tablets as a treatment for hot flashes. The drugs made me feel excellent so I kept taking them until finding my tumor. Now, I know with great certainty that these tablets were the main villain in sparking my unwanted health adventure.

My mind lacks any doubt about this, my soul and heart instinctively convinced of this undeniable truth. We all should listen to our instincts without ignoring them, particularly in matters involving the body.

When asking each of the physicians that I've seen in the past year about the likely cause of my cancer, each identified the conjugated estrogen as the likely cause. But they either would or could not confirm this.

As soon as I stopped using the tablets my youthful skin and vibrant hair suddenly disappeared, while the sweats and hot flashes resumed. This understandably depressed me, since until that point I had always looked younger than my age.

I began thinking, "Oh, well, some sagging skin and lost muscle tone is a price to pay now, better than cancer."

Natural hormone balance must be carefully administered. Doctor Milne keeps mine in check.

Tests proved what I already knew, that my energy and good health had returned. I was up for anything, and still am.

A huge fan of independent films, Jamie still lives in Hollywood, giving her relatively easy access to various movie festivals.

Glad at seeing my steady improvements, one day she gently asked me: "Would you like to go with to me to a film festival? I mean, no big deal if you can't or don't feel up to it. But if you'd like, I'd love to have you as my date."

I smiled at her attempts to avoid pressuring me, still striving to make me as comfortable as possible both emotionally and physically.

"Jamie, I'd love to." I smiled confidently while nodding. "I'll just have to find something to wear."

We joked that moths would fly out of my closet, following my many months of striving to stay as comfortable and casual as possible.

Resuming a regular lifestyle sent energized tendrils of excitement shooting through my entire being, grateful to have emerged as among those who survive such cancer. From this point forward I vowed never to take my life for granted.

A short while later, as Jamie and I sat outside in the California dusk, we crossed paths with many people from her industry. She introduced me and they shook my hand every so delicately as if nervous that a mere touch might crumble my body into dust.

Bright, shining smiles beamed heartily from their startled faces when I heartily squeezed their hands.

"You look great, Ms. Warren," they said. "But are you doing okay?"

My heart and soul never would have wanted anyone to bend down, worriedly asking if I felt okay. I never pitied myself and neither should they.

A realization gently touched the essence of my heart and my physical being as we all talked and laughed, our faces glowing thanks to the radiant orange sunset.

I wouldn't change a thing.

Was the experience terrifying?

Yes, of course. Yet I learned so much, and knowledge is the most valuable lesson we can attain. Especially if my arduous journey had been worthwhile, my experience can be used as a springboard to enable anyone to think outside the box in order to survive cancer.

With each breath that I take today, I remain eternally grateful that my quest to conquer cancer prevailed. You can consider me one of those "lucky ones" who survived, while millions of others lose their battles against this wicked disease each year.

If anyone suffering from cancer today were to ask me for advice, I'd empathically tell them to "stay away from standard doctors, unless absolutely necessary! If you want to live, go natural with IPT chemo—because effective non-poisonous remedies exist."

Just as important, all of us should remember that the mainstream medical industry is flat-out wicked—or purely selfish at the very least—when insisting on unnecessarily using standard chemo and radiation for the treatment of virtually all advance-stage cancers

For the vast majority of people, deep down our hearts command us to live as long as possible, while also striving to maintain good health.

With this understood, allow me to humbly say here that everyone with advance-stage cancer should seek out natural alternative treatments. To do otherwise would be to cave in to the warped thinking of mainstream medicine.

Yes, remember when I found myself nearly on the verge of allowing a Las Vegas clinic to unnecessary subject me to high-dose, extremely toxic chemo that likely would have resulted in my death.

The vast majority of cancer patients want to "be good" and thereby follow their oncologist's every command. Yet in my case my heart and my soul—coupled with common sense—told the essence of my physical being that "something is very wrong."

As you might recall, those sensations had motivated me to suddenly bolt from the clinic of a standard-medicine oncologist. In a round-about way, this was at least to some degree similar to when I had darted as fast as possible from my alcoholic mother's home during my early teens.

Back then I learned that following our common sense and "gut instincts" can lead to survival, or at the very least protection against unnecessary physical harm.

With this understood, consider these questions: "What is your own particular situation today, especially if you or a loved one is now suffering from advancing cancer? What does your heart tell you? Do standard chemo and radiation options strike your mind as seeming illogical? And if you or a relative is being told that 'these treatments are standard,' do you feel as if you're being talked down to—when in fact there might be a better answer?"

In my case, I give credit to following my heart, which always guided me away from what deep down struck me as "wrong"— while also gravitating my body and mind toward everything that felt or seemed "right."

I also emerged from that health scare as a changed person. The experience super-energized my passion to help others battling cancer.

Until my dying day, hopefully at a very advanced age well

past 90, I'll do everything that I reasonably can to help teach people that "unnecessary toxic treatments are the worst way to go."

Long after I'm gone from this earth, if anyone might still remember me, hopefully people will realize that my two greatest passions during the final decades of life were my eternal love for my daughter and the shining need to tell the entire world that there is a fantastic way to live—and that's "the natural way."

Far too often both individually and collectively as a society we put doctors on a pedestal. Still embracing the valuable lessons that I had first learned as a teen, I realize that healthcare is a business just like almost any other money-making venture.

So, look for doctors that refrain from treating you like a number. Make sure they listen to you.

Never fail to seek a second opinion.

All along, remember that no one can make you do anything.

Most important, look for answers—even within yourself.

With just as much urgency, listen to your instincts, which could save your life.

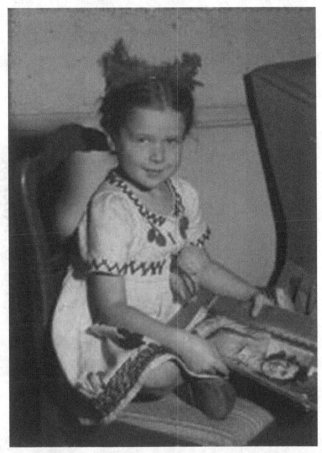

Me at age six by famed Max Factor photographer David Kovar at the Gardian Hotel in Hollywood.

The Gleason Sanitarium—50th Year Anniversary

June 1, 1852, The Gleason Sanitarium (then called The Elmira Water Cure) was opened to the public at Elmira, N. Y., by Drs. S. O. and Rachel B. Gleason, and since that time has been continuously conducted by the Gleason family.

The Sanitarium offers an ideal summer home for those desiring the comforts of a family hotel where the services of a resident physician can be had if necessary. All forms of baths, electricity, and massage are furnished. Modern conveniences. Elevation 1,000 feet. Beautiful and healthful country. Fine drives. Pure spring water. Milk and cream from our own dairy.

Guests received desiring board and medical attention or as boarders only. Write for illustrated booklet to   EDWARD B. GLEASON, Proprietor,

DR. JOHN C. FISHER, *Resident Physician.*   Elmira, N. Y.

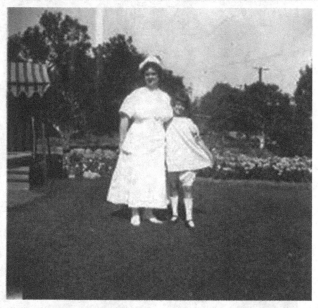

Grandmother Allie & Mother at their Rest Home in Glendale CA. (year unknown)

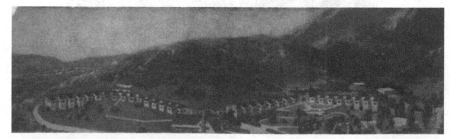

The old Spreckles Hunting Lodge foreground, later became Hillcrest Sanitarium then Pine Tree Lodge, La Cresenta, CA

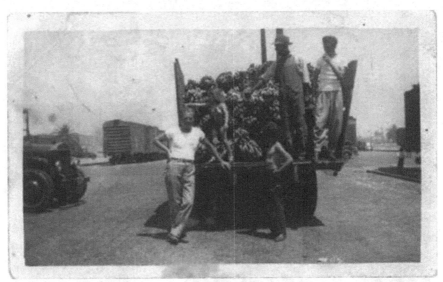

Sol, Me, Bernie or Gen Gelson at Central Market

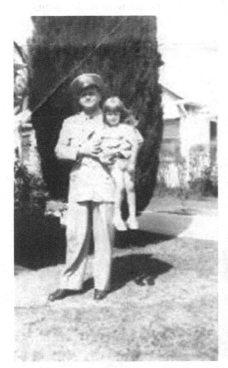

*Last visit with my Father
(1941) until my teens*

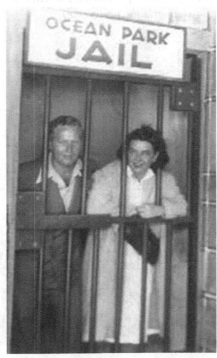

*Sol (new suitor) & Mother late night
at Venice Beach*

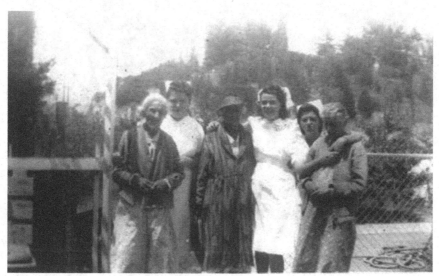

Mother & Father purchased Mt. Gleason Sanitarium. Home with patients and staff. (Mother is the pretty one).

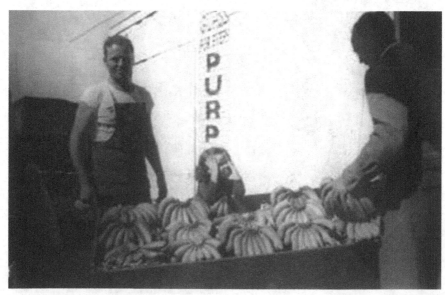

Sol, me & Gene Gelson at our banana stand in Burbank, CA. (year unknown)

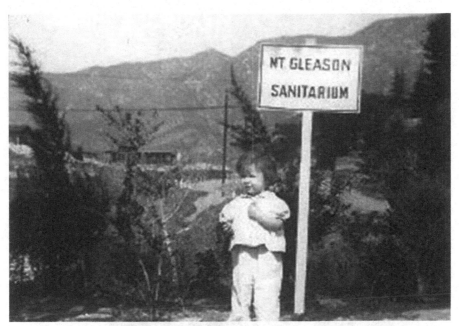

Me playing at the sign and gate entrance. (year unknown)

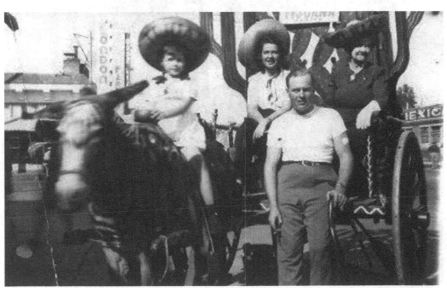

Tijuana Mexico with Sol, me, Mother & Grandmother one of many visits.

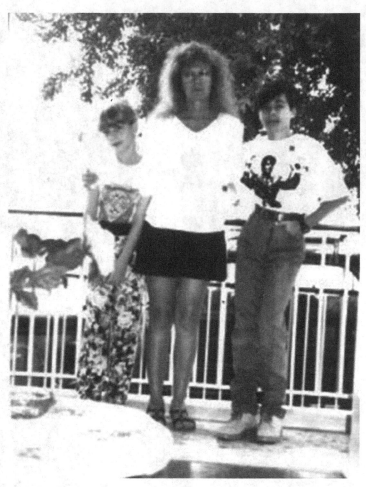

Me in Greece working at film festivals in Europe. (1980's)

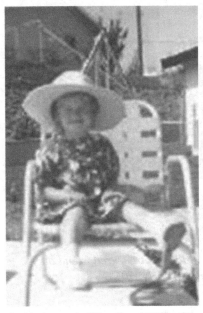
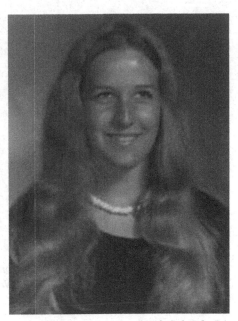

Jamie home in Woodland Hills, CA   *Jamie in Agoura High School, CA*

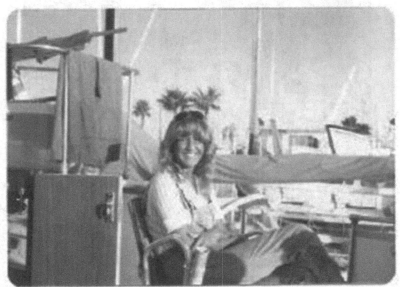

Jamie at Redondo Beach, CA.

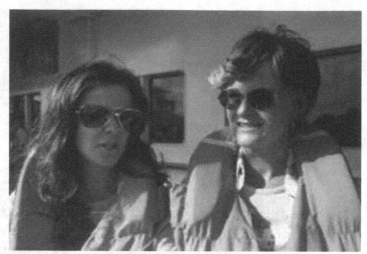

Me and Sharon Riddle my treasured friend on
The Song of Norway.(early '70's)

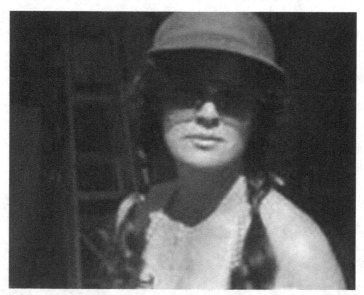

Frank and I building house in Agoura, CA 1984

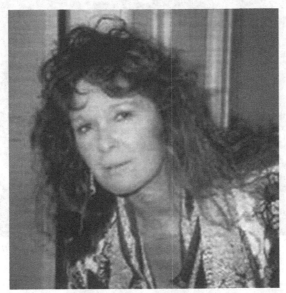

Christmas at friends home 1980s

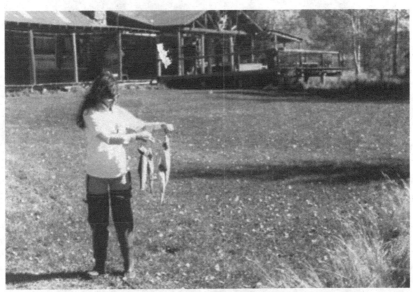

My string of Brookies, Henry's Lake Idaho 1980s

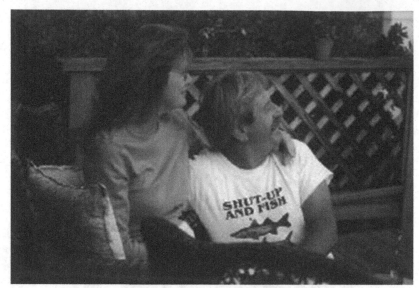

Me & Frank, he was a great nurse (2003)

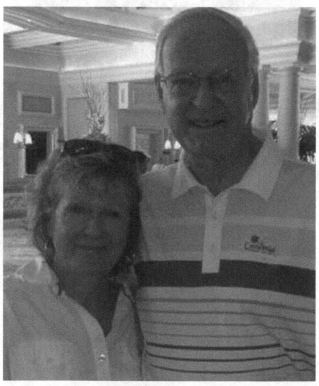

Me and Jamie's Father after my cancer

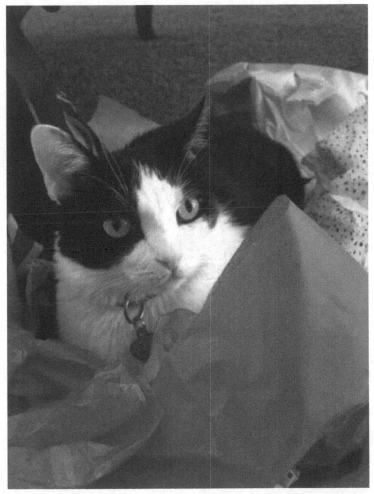

Ken stops snuggling

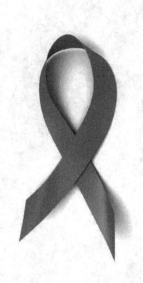

Part 11
Alternatives and Health Maintenance

Chapter 1
You Are What You Eat

Earning millions of dollars daily, the giant health care industry firmly keeps "standard of care" rules in place. Big bucks keep rolling in hour after hour as the many forlorn growing masses of people suffer diminishing bodies and rampant cancer.

The bottom line is that no one will take action against the complacent status quo until enough people get angry at the degeneration of integrity and logic in our country. To inspire change many people must express their dissatisfaction with the status quo. Otherwise, the critical effort for necessary change will fail.

Why do we not use the Greece test first and foremost?

Shouldn't health care stand for winning, working and fighting for truth and not just "searching" for apparent, possible "cures" while many effective remedies actually are already available to us?

Saying that we can now cure all cancer would be irresponsible. Yet effective non-toxic and non-poisonous remedies exist, and in many instances such effective treatments could be used perfectly in conjunction with criteria stipulated in each specific Greece test.

Strangely and to the great detriment of society as a whole,

many doctors fear going outside the "standard of care" dictated by the USA's mainstream medical industry.

This is not to imply or to unequivocally state that that dangerous radiation and highly toxic chemo levels ultimately fail in 100-percent of cancer cases.

But please examine the numbers. As mentioned earlier, if I randomly grouped five people that I know, at least one of them would have some type of cancer during his or her lifetime. This widespread occurrence is worth analyzing.

The per-capita instances of cancer are significantly lower in East African and Mediterranean countries than in the United States and Western cultures. This ignites an urgent need to evaluate our own lifestyle

Look at the foods we eat!
Look at the products we use!
Look at the products in our businesses and homes!
Look at the chemical trails that ruin our clear blue skies and water supplies!

We should always remain aware of what accumulates in our bodies. Look at the huge number of drugs that have dangerous and horrible side effects.

Our society and the medical profession as a whole each need to do a much better job tracking and quantifying the dangers of radiation and chemo.

Unlike streams of helpful and effective natural, non-toxic remedies, the standard chemo and radiation treatments inherently generate adverse and sometimes fatal reactions—killing good cells while wrecking or destroying natural bodily defenses.

The same goes for mainstream high-priced drugs made by the gigantic pharmaceutical industry. Many prescription drugs ranging from sleep remedies to pain suppressants cause far more problems than they solve.

Examine and Revolutionize Your Diet

Support doctors that listen, search and have open minds, while also courageous enough to support organic foods, supplements, the no-sugar diet approach, good weight and natural food alternatives. Here is a list to help you navigate the grocery store aisles, putting you on tracking for making optimal decisions to achieve lasting good health.

- Dairy, wheat and corn cause physical disorders among many people. Lots of individuals are allergic to dairy without knowing this. Do you have a "sore" or funny feeling in your stomach after eating wheat cereal with milk, perhaps even worsened by orange juice? None of those foods make for a happy stomach. The combination can cause gas and bloating. Non-wheat cereals also may cause this; you have to experiment with your food combinations and identify triggers. This is because gluten in cereals is often harsher on the stomach along with lactose. Easier to digest, goat milk is a delicious alternative for cow's-milk sensitive people.

- Go vegan, except for organic meats and poultry to give your body the best quality food. Think of your body as a vehicle. It takes you from point A to point B. Knowledgeable personnel at many car facilities refuse to put bad or cheap gas in their cars because such fuel fails to enable the car to run as smoothly as possible. This equates to the way foods that we choose impacts our bodies. Why would a person eat anything but the healthiest and highest quality meals? Are we not worth that? After all, our bodies are the most important vehicles.

- Avoid farm fish, which tend to contain dangerously high toxin levels, while larger fish tend to have dangerously high mercury levels. According to the Environmental protection agency, often called the EPA, excessive and dangerous mercury levels have been shown to cause tumors in lab rats. Typically untainted by toxins, Himalayan salt such be the only type of

131

salt in our diets. Toxic pollutants contaminate ocean water, making "sea salt" much less desirable. Scientists say that Himalayan salt contains all 84 of the natural minerals and elements found in the human body. In addition to regulating pH, this substance facilitates optimal water balance and healthy urination and bowel movements. Meantime, Himalayan salt improves sinus and vascular health, while reducing the risk of kidney stones, rheumatism and other health issues, especially beneficial when trying to lose weight. Himalayan salt also reduces the appearance of cellulite. Our bodies have difficulty metabolizing table salt, which becomes harmful sodium chloride when processed by the body.

- CALM relaxing powder has many benefits, simple to mix in water and drink during the day.
- Green tea, brown tea and black teas are all good for us. Drink them warm or cold, and purchase only organic name brands. The antioxidants in green tea, for example, help prevent development of cancer of the breast, lung, pancreas and other vital organs. Black tea reduces the risk of stroke, while also having protective properties for people whose lungs have been exposed to secondhand smoke.

The benefits of Himalayan salt, published on May 15, 2009, by Dr. Edward F. Group II, DC.

Types of Teas and their Health Benefits, By Julie Edgar, WebMD feature reviewed by Louise Chang, M.D., accessed February 5, 2013.

- Goat products like milk, butter, yogurt—especially the yummy apricot—provide a pleasant change for people allergic to dairy cow milk
- Nuts: Eat seeds, walnuts, pecans, brazils, or almonds

daily, unsalted unless seasoned with Himalayan salt.
- Uli Mana, a raw cacao treat, can be purchased via the Internet if you want to avoid sugar but love chocolate. Some Whole Foods stores carry a few of these products, but this conglomerate's Website offers the best selection.
- Stevia is a healthy, natural, minimal-calorie sweetener.
- Xylitol looks and tastes the same as regular white sugar but only has about one third less calories than table sugar, according to various published reports. Bake and sprinkle Xylitol on anything for which you would use regular sugar.

Maintain a Balanced pH

Keep your pH in balance. Many pharmacies sell testing kits. This one measure can benefit your body in a big way. Just drinking a little club soda each day will help balance your pH. Adding several drops of lemon juice to your orange juice makes the beverage alkaline, preventing acid reactions.

Why does pH matter?

Cancer thrives in acidic biological environments. Indeed, your pH balance is critical for your immune system, particularly when suffering from illness. Many germs and bacteria die or fail to grow in a balanced pH environment, while thriving and posing extreme health threats when in acidic conditions.

Certain foods can generate a dangerous acidic environment. Many peoples' bodies become increasingly acidic as they age, particularly into the senior years. As mentioned earlier, sugar often thrives in acidic conditions, fueling cancer and any growth of the disease. You can use the Internet to identify acidic or acid-generating foods and adjust your diet accordingly. Death can result when the body becomes unable to naturally reverse an overly acidic environment.

Under normal conditions people almost never experience issues with their pH balance. But haywire pH levels increase the probability that you'll develop an illness such as a cold sore, a sore throat or a much more serious ailment like cancer. Then again, an out-of-whack pH system might never even bother you.

If you're interested in what your pH balance reading is, at most pharmacies you can purchase measurement sticks for determining those levels within saliva or urine.

The Liver

As doctor Mehmet Oz says, "The first thing in the morning take a glass with a small amount of warm water, add a few drops of lemon juice and four or five drops of Tobasco Sauce™ and drink." Your liver will be happy because in the morning your system is clear enough to where the water can more easily cleanse the organ, flush through your system, become absorbed and as a healthful result, burn more calories and clear your complexion.

Chapter 2
DCA and Haelan 951

DCA

Dichloroacetic acid, abbreviated as DCA, is the compound with the chemical formula $CHCl_2COOH$. During in-vitro and animal studies, DCA has shown to reduce tumors, although there is no substantial evidence that it helps humans during cancer treatment.

In spite of the so-called lack of evidence, there have been many successful studies. For example, the University of Alberta conducted a study on DCA in 2007 in which they applied DCA on cancer cells from a human that was grown in mice. * During this research, DCA revived the function of the cell's mitochondria. This in turn allows for apoptosis (programmed cell death), allowing cancer cells to self-destruct and shrink the tumor.*

* "Cheap, 'safe' drug kills most cancers" New Scientist. 2007-01-17. Retrieved 2007-01-17.

* Bonnet, Sébastien; Archer, Stephen L.; Allalunis-Turner, Joan; Haromy, Alois; Beaulieu, Christian; Thompson, Richard; Lee, Christopher T.; Lopaschuk, Gary D. et al. (2007). "A Mitochondria-K+ Channel Axis Is Suppressed in Cancer and Its Normalization Promotes Apoptosis and Inhibits Cancer Growth". *Cancer Cell* **11** (1): 37–51. doi:10.1016/j.ccr.2006.10.020. PMID 17222789

The New Scientist magazine describes this phenomenon as switching off the cancer cells' immortality. This is important for the reason listed below, courtesy of the DCA Site:

"A non-cancerous cell will initiate apoptosis when it detects damage within itself that it cannot repair. But a cancer cell resists the suicide process. That is why chemotherapy and radiation treatments do not work very well and actually result in terrible side effects … the healthy cells actually die much easier." *

Unfortunately, much of the support of DCA comes from other countries. The United States still clings to chemo and radiation in its standard of care. No studies have been conducted in the United States just yet, although it is gaining momentum as the public becomes increasingly interested due to media coverage.

* The DCA Site, "DCA and How It Works." Last modified 2007-2010. Accessed March 15, 2013. http://www.thedcasite.com/dca_how_it_works.html.

Haelan 951

Haelan 951 is the fermented soybean beverage that I mentioned. Its healing properties come from the soybean's isoflavones. German researchers have found that this component of the soybean stops growth of tumors and helps fend off cancer. One of the most potent isoflavones is called genistein, which has a wide array of benefits:

1. As with other isoflavones, acts as an anti-estrogen by blocking the uptake of estrogen;

3. Inhibits other enzymes involved in cancer progression;

4. Causes cancer cells to differentiate and change back to normal cells. A normal cell becomes cancerous by de-differentiating – in other words becoming more embryonic (primitive) or less specialized, and therefore more deadly. Genistein reverses this process; *

An additional miraculous attribute of Haelan 951 occurs thanks to its unique ability to prevent the ingrowth of potentially dangerous capillaries. When left unchecked, such blood vessels help enable malignant tumors to spread by nourishing cancerous cells. Haelan 951 inhibits that process by effectively blocking the nourishment which otherwise would enable tumors to thrive. While also serving as an anti-oxidant, Haelan 951 inhibits angiogenesis, thereby resulting in cancer cell death due to starvation.

*Excerpt from the following publication: Isoflavones and the New Concentrated Soy Supplements by Phillip N. Steinberg, Certified Nutritional Consultant, graduate of the Nutritionists Institute of America. Copyright 1996.

It's interesting that in countries where soy (not GMO) is a diet staple, primarily in Asian countries, women see much fewer instances of breast cancer as they're at lower risk.

Haelan 951 is so effective because fermenting the soybean hydrolyzes the soy to where we get these invaluable proteins and genistein. The product itself was developed for the purpose of providing the most nutritional value to patients. It also boosts the immune system during the pivotal breast cancer battle. Haelan 951 uses the best soybeans on the market – soybeans are more potent depending on the age and type.*

Using it has been shown in studies to block off the pathways allowing cancer cells to mutate and grow.

As the man who sells me the Haelan says, because their research involves a complex nutritional product that falls in the "food" category, the FDA does not allow disease claims or advertisements for products without extensive expensive clinical studies to establish safety and efficacy. Therefore, the fermented soy has not had the exposure it should have.

In addition, most people believe soy phytoestrogens are estrogens, make cancers grow quicker and increase feminine characteristics in men. Studies show none of this is true. In this area I would like to point out the fact that a highly successful PTSD study using Haelan 951 showed the Haelan 951 soy formulation doubled the testosterone levels of young Elite NATO military soldiers suffering from PTSD, which brought them up to normal testosterone levels. Soy phytoestrogens are not estrogenic and are in fact anti-estrogenic. In addition, they have very effective anti-

* Haelan Products, "History of Haelan 851." Last modified 2002. Accessed March 15, 1013. http://haelanproducts.com/history.htm.

cancer properties and many beneficial mechanisms of action for the cancer patient. *

They say that getting pregnant in your youth can reduce breast cancer risk by fifty percent. Interestingly, the hormones involved in that process and prevention closely resemble soy isoflavones, both having anticancer effects. *

Without delving too deeply in the science of it, Haelan 951 was a key player in my success. Although it tastes like brake fluid, my means of helping improve the taste was a true help and essential to ingesting it as I needed. For more information, look at the Additional Reading section of this book.

* Walter H. Wainwright, President, Haelan Research Foundation

* Rohr, Uwe D., Anca G. Gocan, Doris Bachg, and Adolf E. Schindler. "Cancer protection of soy resembles cancer protection during pregnancy." *Horm Mol Biol Clin Invest.* (2010): n. page. Print.

Chapter 3
Chemo and
the Greek Blood Test

The Revolutionary Chemo

Conventional chemotherapy is notorious for being a grueling, horrific ordeal. Debilitating nausea accompanies flu-like symptoms, such as chills and fevers. Women lose their prized feature, their hair. In addition to killing off the important cells, it damages necessary components of the body such as the immune system.

Because conventional chemotherapy is a blind killer, unable to differentiate between good cells along with the bad, it isn't the most logical option. This affects the blood, often requiring patients to get transfusions, and makes patients more susceptible to illness in their already weakened state. If only we could take the good of chemotherapy and eliminate the adverse side effects, right?

Insulin Potentiation Therapy (IPT)

But there is an answer. There is a chemotherapy called Insulin Potentiation Therapy (IPT). IPT utilizes our newfound knowledge of cells in this modern age.

IPT treatment (low dose targeted chemotherapy) is a conventional cancer treatment with a modification that not only solves the above problems, but also provides a kinder and gentler way to treat cancer with fewer negative side effects. IPT treatment for cancer can be considered simply as chemotherapy, but a more refined and gentler style of chemotherapy.

But what are the benefits of such a treatment?

IPT chemo, unlike its predecessor, doesn't take that much of a toll on the patient. However, it successfully differentiates between cells only killing the cancer. This is important because in any tumor 99.1 percent to 99.9 percent of the cells in the original tumor are non-malignant cancer cells. These do not hurt people unless space is limited, like in the brain, and they can't spread to vital organs. Chemotherapy and radiation do not kill cancer stem cells; they only selectively kill the non-malignant cells in the tumor.

In addition, chemotherapy blocks cell differentiation and increases the numbers of cancer stem cells that are treatment resistant with conventional chemotherapy and/or radiation treatments. This is why the death rate from metastatic cancer has not dropped in the last thirty years. (This was published in Cancer Research in 2006 and confirmed by Dr. Max Wicha, University of Michigan stem cell expert.)

It certainly has its critics, but it's good to keep in mind that the procedure is done carefully and methodically. As with anything, the procedure has been improved from the first trials and implementations. Also, if you were a diabetic, you might need extra care. A well-trained staff of plenty of nurses is required in order to monitor each person carefully. If that is not in place, then one should not seek treatment at that facility!

Your hair may thin, but by taking the biotin-forte it comes back thicker. I never felt bad after the treatments. You need to follow directions, rest, eat properly and remain positive. I had six treatments within three weeks. I stayed near the Wellness Clinic in Reno and went home on the weekends. My support was the Whole Foods Market, suggested health food restaurants, friendly taxi drivers. Many hotels give discounts when you are attending the therapy clinics too, so that's an added bonus.

In my experience I was closely monitored to where my blood sugar was so low I became slightly light headed. Right before that point the cancer cells went out to gobble up the sugar I ingested and were destroyed by the (IV) injection. This requires only ten percent of the amount of chemo used in other chemotherapy methods. I'm no expert but that sounds efficient to me. Add the fact that it's only a couple hours per week, much cheaper and the fact it has caused no deaths!

Cancer Chemosensitivity Testing

Doctor Forsythe explains the important Greek Test in detail, as seen here from the October 2010 Century Wellness Clinic Newsletter. You should read his entire article. I am sure this will help you to form an opinion regarding the Greek Test, an essential step during the initial diagnosis process.

WELLNESS MONTHLY

October 2010

Cutting Edge Technology....
Gene Testing has the Answers
By Dr. James W. Forsythe

Monthly Newsletter
Century Wellness Clinic

521 Hammill Lane
Reno, Nevada 89511
775-827-0707
drForsythe.com
centurywellness@gmail.com

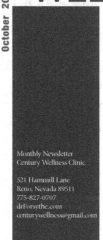

"No other oncologist in the United States can offer this kind of information to his or her patients. What conventional oncologists offer only is what has been the best results of the latest clinical study."

-Dr. James W. Forsyth

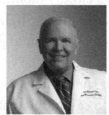

Cancer Chemosensitivity Testing in my mind after 40 years of practicing cancer medicine is the biggest "C Change" that I have seen in all my years of practice with over 200,000 patient visits. The advent of Cancer Chemosensitivity Testing in our practice has made a major difference in the lives of our patients' success rates and improved overall survival rates. These statistics show up in our current 5 -Year, 500 patient study. This study using various combinations of conventional and natural therapies in what is termed as the overall designation of Integrative Oncology.

Let me explain how the testing is done at Century Wellness Clinic.... Some people come to me as virginal treatment patients, who have had no treatments at all or have had multiple drug, radiation, chemotherapy or perhaps even surgery to start with. They are in situations where their disease is progressing. Most patients are Stage IV cancers. All patients are seeking answers. They know their disease is advancing and their prognosis is guarded. They know their time factors are limited and they want real answers.

They don't want a guessing game and they don't want an oncologist that picks out drugs and throws them against a wall to see if any stick in terms of their own cancer response rates.

What we do and tell the patent is .... You have to rely on the test by taking the whole blood from the patient. This testing is a very easy sample to obtain. The blood is then handled very carefully, with special packaging and shipping requirements . The blood is drawn at the first part of the week in order to get it to its' destination in a safe, preserved and fresh manner. The blood is then subjected to very high technology testing. There are four labs in the world that do this testing that we are aware of - Two in Germany, one in Greece and one in South Korea. We have found that the Greek test offers the most important information in terms of the number of chemotherapy agents tested, as well as the number of supplements tested. In fact the Greek test (RGCC, Research Genetic Cancer Center) tests 18 families of chemotherapy agents and 38 families of supplements. Once they have the blood, it takes anywhere from ten days to three weeks to analyze the sample and harvest the gene cells from the blood and break them genetically to determine the gene markers. These gene markers are compared with what various chemotherapy agents do in relationship with these markers and from this information they are able to tell which drugs work the best

Cont. on back page

Winning my Battle Against Stage 2 Breast Cancer

Cont. from front page

out of the 18 and which supplements out of the 38 work the best. They send a full report back to me. I then sit down with the patient, draw up a formula that marries both the conventional drugs and the best supplements into a protocol which then becomes the patient's own genetic blueprint. This is a very specific and definitive test. No other oncologist in the United States can offer this kind of information to his or her patients. What conventional oncologists offer only is what has been the best results of the latest clinical study. These studies are not 100% accurate. Many are only 30%, 40%, or 50% accurate. Results will show that one half to two thirds of patients would not be helped by chemotherapy. These patients would merely be poisoned if given chemotherapy, which would do nothing to eliminate their cancer. These drugs are cellular toxins causing either chemo-brain syndrome, cardiac toxicities, peripheral neuropathies, bone marrow suppression to severe generalized rashes. The ultimate toxicity is death. It is not unusual for patients after a severe bout of chemotherapy to experience adverse side affects.

Once we marry the protocol together, I recommend low dose-fractionated insulin potentiated therapy as my first choice. If the patient wishes to go conventional, they at least know what are the best drugs for them. At that point, they then have the right answer. They can either be treated by me or preferentially go home and be treated by their local oncologist. We also send them home with the appropriate supplements that are very effective against their cancer. We renew their supplements on a monthly basis.

The real value of the Cancer Chemosensitivity Testing in my practice has accounted for a higher response rate to the therapy I now give to my patients.

Meet your team..
Manon Niel, L.P.N.

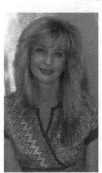

Manon Is a Licensed Practical Nurse who has been working in the medical industry for over 20 years. She has been Dr. Forsythe's infusion room nurse for more than 12 years. Patients have confidence and trust in her skills and abilities. Manon administers fractionated chemotherapy with insulin potentiated therapy (IPT). She also makes complementary IVs under the direction of Dr. Forsythe that are specific to every patient. Each individual receives an immune booster or Forsythe Immune Treatment (FIT). These customized immune boosters (FIT) promote the immune system to fight the individuals' cancer. Along with the (FIT) and the Cancer Chemosensitivity Test, the protocol to conquer ones' cancer is realized.

Manon Niel

Suzanne Somers
Blog
By Suzanne Somers

In KNOCKOUT, Dr. James Forsythe explains that in both Germany and Greece, specialists begin by harvesting the cancer cells out of the patient's blood. They then break down the cells genetically in order to discover which markers are compatible with treatment of the tumor. From this, they can tell which drugs would be most effective for the particular cancer, which ones would be ineffective, or harmful. Once the correct type of chemo has been determined, Dr. Forsythe uses an integrative treatment, with far lower doses of chemo (10-20% of the norm), far fewer side effects, and much better results.

Read more about Dr. Forsythe on Suzanne's blog at

suzannesomers.com Blog ChemosensitivityTest Why Does Big Pharma Know About Them and We Dont

My Greek Blood Test

For your review, I've included here an actual copy of results of my personal Greek Test. As you can clearly see, the findings designate which potential treatments are most effective for each patient's particular type of cancer. Just as essential, the results of the Greek Test also specify which possible treatments would most likely fail to eradicate the individual's cancer. This emerges as a vital phase, since Greek Test results in some specific instances can "rule out" any perceived need to take highly toxic, potentially deadly "standard-of-care" high dose chemo and radiation. As previously stated, the results of my personal test essentially "saved my life," specifying that high-dose chemo would have emerged as an unnecessary and potentially deadly treatment in my case.

My Investigated Supplements

These are some of the supplements I have taken and investigated. Most are for the body's immune system but not "proven" to help:

Chloroxygen – says it builds red blood cells

Black currant oil

Biotin didn't work for me; only the biotin-forte made my hair thick

Pau D'arco

Green Tea Leaf extract – immune support

De aromatase (in my case, it did nothing)

ImmunePower

Red clover extract

Celery seed extract

PectaSol-C – modified citrus pectin

Host defense

Iodoral

BAM – a vitamin (really hard to swallow)

BioSil – nails and hair strengthener. Again, in my case the biotin forte made my hair thicker.

Super Lysine – for me it prevents and aids in curing infection.

Aloe ease

Genistein soy complex – for upset stomach.

Grady's DETOX

Bata 1,3D Glucan

Carnivora – terrific. For me it assisted with energy, but not as well as the Haelan 951 did.

Super Bio – Cucumin

Life Shield Immunity – mushrooms defense

Hoxsey's clover burdock

True food super-potency soyagen

Evening primrose oil

Carnivora lymph drainage

Indole-3 – carbinol

Gavio-cat – graviola and cat's claw

Milk thistle – if you have hemochromatosis, you should avoid this.

LifeOne – high in iron

C-statin

DIMension 3

Taurine

Vitamin K2 – helped me with severe bruising

Rejeneril

Poly 3

Quercetin

Alpha-Lipoic Acid

Lglutathione

Detoxygen

Papaya Enzyme – for digestion

Dr. Robert D. Milne's book PC Liposomal Encapsulation Technology (or LET) has valuable information. The subject is defined as "Proven nano-chemistry that can make health and longevity supplements many times more efficient and effective." "Liposomal encapsulation protects substances from most of the degrading and inhibitory factors (such as the use of binders for tablets, capsules, coatings, artificial colors, artificial flavors, sugar and other additives that can diminish the digestibility and uptake of nutrients and therapeutic substances). It provides an unparalleled payload protection."

"LET utilizes phospholipid litposomes to form a barrier around their contents that is resistant to digestive juices, alkaline solutions and salts found in the human body as well as free radicals. Because of this, they do a superior job in protecting the contents from oxidation and degradation from external substances and conditions.".

"Most importantly, this protective barrier stays intact until the contents have been delivered to the gland, organ or system where the contents will be used."

All the studies and research regarding the use of essential phospholipids and phosphatidylcholine (PC) cited in his book were accomplished using polyunsaturated PC

Some of the benefits include:
Reduction in total serum lipids—fat in the blood
Reduction in LDL—bad cholesterol
Increase in HDL—good cholesterol
Reduction in total cholesterol
Reduction in triglycerides
Reduction in cholesterol deposits in vascular walls

Reduction in blood platelet aggregation (detrimental tendency of blood cells to stick together)
Effective antioxidants in lipids
Increased coronary circulation
Increased exercise tolerance
Improved peripheral circulation (hand and feet)
Liver protection and rejuvenation
Improved immunity
Improved memory
Prevention of excess collagen formation and cross-linking (wrinkles and scarring)

Personally, I take the C and glutathione and have seen vast improvements since beginning to intake it on a daily basis. One bottle, the larger one, is tasty and I take one teaspoon per day. The smaller bottle doesn't taste bad, just bland. I take a little less than a teaspoon each day, both about fifteen minutes before a meal.

I tend to have high blood pressure but that has since gone down. Bruising had been a big problem the past three years, but that has also since improved greatly. I have more energy, improved skin, I sleep better and it's so easy to take! There is much more detailed information in Dr. Milne's little booklet that is useful for each individual's needs.

Regarding cancer, my successes were with the healing and energy-giving Haelan 951 and DCA. Plenty of C, glutathione, D3, and other vitamins have made my immune system strong. The supplements listed on the Greece test provided by Dr. Forsythe (except for DCA) were critical in my overall recovery.

Don't forget that eating correctly is the major key to health. I've always eaten healthy since college, but now since having cancer I have learned how immeasurably important it really is. Read labels, search the Internet, find out what you are allergic to, and go organic.

Again, it's worth the effort. You must work to find what is best for your particular body. We are all so different and what works for one doesn't work for others. Now on occasion I walk into a big super market just to purchase salt for my water softener. I look around at the enormous number of chemicals, pre-packaged foods, frozen, diet foods, canned chemicals, hormone-treated meats, farmed fish, chicken that has been fed who knows what and vegetables that are shipped from everywhere except local farmers and sprayed with pesticides that are toxic if inhaled, let alone eaten. It's no wonder that almost one out of five people we know has cancer or some similar illness. Cancer treatment centers are bursting with patients. Radiation could be okay for very localized cancers, but I still feel that we must try finding what fits our personal consciences and what is logical.

If you have to stay up late or get up early, read up on all you can find about your specific condition. There is a vast amount of knowledge on the Internet, books and you need to investigate beyond the Standard of Care. The world is full of information we don't see or hear about in our everyday medical "news". It's knowing what is out there and studying continually so you can work with logical doctors and solutions. Have an open mind and don't be afraid to go to other doctors for opinions. If you have to pay out of your own pocketbook for opinions that are not supported by your insurance, then do it! Sell a television, a car, move to a smaller, less inexpensive home or apartment but make the investment in yourself. Always question why the treatment is so many weeks, why is the chemo such a high dose, why? Why? Why? Understand what it will do to you in the long run. Build up your body with the right vitamins, healthy diet and supplements that are suggested to help your immune system fight for your life and good health.

It's a constant battle. Cancer never takes a holiday!

Additional Reading

http://www.drforsythe.com

http://www.terinomd.com/meetdrterino.html

http://www.vitals.com/doctors/Dr_John_Matrisciano.html

http://www.youtube.com/watch?v=prtRcOuzJCY

http://www.haelanproducts.com

http://www.rgcc-genlab.com

http://www.iptq.com

PC LIPOSOMAL ENCAPSULATION TECHNOLOGY
by Dr. Robert D. Milne M.D.

Knockout by Suzanne Somers

To Contact Diana Warren
merchantbank@earthlink.net
ForeverMediaPublishing.com

TRUE DIRECTIONS
An affiliate of Tarcher Books

OUR MISSION

Tarcher's mission has always been to publish books
that contain great ideas. Why? Because:

GREAT LIVES BEGIN WITH GREAT IDEAS

At Tarcher, we recognize that many talented authors, speakers,
educators, and thought-leaders share this mission and deserve to be
published – many more than Tarcher can reasonably publish ourselves.
True Directions is ideal for authors and books that increase awareness,
raise consciousness, and inspire others to live their ideals and passions.

Like Tarcher, True Directions books are designed to do three things:
inspire, inform, and motivate.

Thus, True Directions is an ideal way for these important voices to
bring their messages of hope, healing, and help to the world.

Every book published by True Directions– whether it is non-fiction, memoir,
novel, poetry or children's book – continues Tarcher's mission to publish works
that bring positive change in the world. We invite you to join our mission.

For more information, see the True Directions website:
www.iUniverse.com/TrueDirections/SignUp

Be a part of Tarcher's community to bring positive change in this world!
See exclusive author videos, discover new and exciting books, learn about
upcoming events, connect with author blogs and websites, and more!
www.tarcherbooks.com

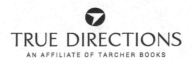

TRUE DIRECTIONS
AN AFFILIATE OF TARCHER BOOKS